STROKE RECOVERY

WHAT NOW?
When Physical Therapy Ends,
But Your Recovery Continues

By

Tracy L. Markley, C.P.T
Fitness & Biomechanics Specialist

Dedicated to

All Stroke Survivors

Never Give Up!

TABLE OF CONTENTS

INTRODUCTION

This book is written for stroke survivors, caregivers, physical therapists, fitness professionals and all who are helping a stroke survivor either personally or professionally. I came to write about stroke recovery after I had a unique and special experience training a 65-year-old stroke survivor almost every day for over two years. He was an excellent example of what great recovery gains can come if a survivor can move and exercise every day, especially with proper guidance. This led to my first book "A Stoke of An Artist; The Journey of a Fitness Trainer and A Stroke Survivor." After this book was published, I began to be contacted internationally to share more of my knowledge and our story. I began speaking at some stroke recovery support groups, and I found many survivors that have struggled with different challenges to find more therapy or fitness professionals to guide them in continued recovery.

All survivors are recovering at their own unique pace. There are many different levels of damage caused by a stroke. Understand that all survivors will be different and not everything in this book will help all survivors.

I was recently asked to be on the Education Advisory Board for the Medfit Network and to write the Stroke Recovery and Exercise continued education course.

As a fitness professional, I usually meet a stroke recovery client after they have finished their therapy sessions with a physical therapist. Depending on the intensity of the stroke, this can be after a month or up to many months spent in an in-patient care facility, where they receive physical therapy every day and/or only after having out-patient physical therapy.

Both physical therapists and fitness professionals have options to continue to search out the most updated research and knowledge to help them in their work and care with their patients/ clients. They may be required by management where they work to do so, or it is left as a personal decision by individuals in either profession. It is important to understand that when professionals limit continued education, they can limit recovery in a survivor. If a survivor and/or their caregiver do not know any better, they will think all their continued limits are just from their stroke, when in fact it is very possible that they were limited by the limited education of their trainer or therapist. As you continue through this book, you will find there is not a structured step-by-step format for each survivor to follow, since each stroke survivor case is different.

CHAPTER 1

WHAT IS A STROKE?

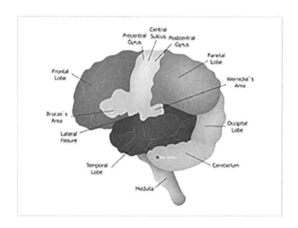

By now I am sure all your medical professionals have answered the question," What is a Stroke?" So I will share briefly for those who may need more understanding. A stroke is damage to the brain by interrupted blood supply. A stroke can also be referred to as a brain attack or a CVA, cerebrovascular accident. This can occur when a clot blocks the blood supply to the brain or when a blood vessel in the brain bursts. A stroke is a medical emergency. Always call 911 or get immediately to the hospital. The longer any stroke is left untreated, the more likely it is that the affected organs can be permanently damaged.

Blood supplies oxygen and nutrients to the brain. When an area of the brain tissue does not receive its blood supply, it results in brain damage. This is known as an infarction or infarct. An infarction can happen anywhere in the body, but in relation to a stroke, it is referring to the blood supply limited in an area of the brain. An infarct can affect a tiny or large part of the brain. Anything that cuts off blood supply to the brain compromises brain function. The neurons in the area of the brain that has been cut off from blood supply begin to die, and the functions they support will be affected. Adult brains make few or no neurons, therefore the biological damage is permanent. Strokes can cause serious motor and cognitive problems and sometimes permanent damage. Recovery depends on the remaining undamaged area of the brain. As in a heart attack, heart tissue dies. In a brain attack, brain tissues die.

Symptoms of stroke include trouble walking, speaking, slurring words and understanding as well as paralysis or numbness of the face, arm or leg.

Identify a stroke by using the **F.A.S.T** test

FACE   Is their face drooping on one side? Can they smile normally?

ARMS   Can they raise both arms and keep them there?

SPEECH (Speaking) Are they slurring in their speech?

TIME   Any signs of a stroke call 911 immediately! Time is brain.

It is crucial to get immediate medical attention with any sign of a stroke, even if it appears to be a mini-stroke.

In an **Ischemic Stroke** (Blockage), if caught within three hours, it can be treated by tPA (Tissue Plasminogen Activator). It is FDA-approved for treatment for ischemic strokes. tPA is found naturally in the body to destroy blood clots. When tPA is promptly given in the limited time frame following a stroke, it can save lives and reduce the long-term effects of stroke. It works to dissolve the clot and improve the blood flow to the part of the brain being deprived of the blood flow. Early treatment with medications like tPA (clot buster) can minimize brain damage. Time can be a determination of a full recovery. Time is brain.

In a **Hemorrhagic Stroke** (Rupture/leak), the treatment goal is to stop the bleeding ASAP. This occurs by surgery to clip or coil an artery to stop the bleeding from spreading farther into or through the brain.

Other treatments focus on limiting complications and preventing additional strokes.

The body has contralateral organization. This means the brain's left hemisphere controls the right side of the body, and the brain's right hemisphere controls the left side of the body. This works even in the "Sensory" as in "Spatial awareness." The right side of the brain controls what we sense in our space around us on the left side of the body as the left side of the brain controls what we sense in our space around us on the right side.

Since research shows that 80% of strokes can be prevented, here are the top 10 things to watch out for from the National Stroke Association. This also means 20% could not have been prevented.

1. Know your blood pressure.

2. Check for AFib (Atrial Fibrillation), AFib or AF is a quivering or irregular heartbeat (arrythmia) that can lead to blood clots, stroke and heart failure.

3. Don't smoke. Smoking doubles the risk of stroke.

4. Drink in moderation.

5. Manage cholesterol.

6. Manage diabetes.

7. Exercise.

8. Low fat and low sodium diet.

9. Watch circulation.

10. Call 911 at any symptoms of a stroke.

If you would like to see statistics, here are a few:

Someone has a stroke every 40 seconds in the United States. Based on the latest statistics by the National Stroke Association (Stroke.org), there are nearly 7 million stroke survivors in the U.S. Stroke is the 5th leading cause of death in the U.S. Stroke can happen to anyone at any time. Twice as many women die from stroke than breast cancer. A stroke can happen at any age.

CHAPTER 2

TYPES OF STROKES

The three main types of stroke are:

- Ischemic Stroke
- Hemorrhagic Stroke
- TIA Transient Ischemic Attack, "mini-stroke," warning sign

Ischemic Stroke

Most strokes are ischemic strokes. According to the Center for Disease Control (CDC), about 87% of strokes are ischemic. An ischemic stroke happens when blood flow through the artery that supplies oxygen-rich blood to the brain becomes blocked.

Blood clots often cause the blockages that lead to ischemic strokes.

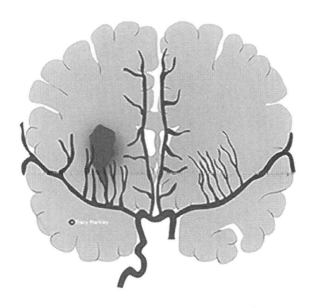

Hemorrhagic Stroke

A hemorrhagic stroke happens when an artery in the brain leaks blood or ruptures (breaks open). The leaked blood puts too much pressure on brain cells, which damages them. High blood pressure and aneurysms, balloon-like bulges, in an artery that can stretch and burst, are examples of conditions that can cause a hemorrhagic stroke.

There are two types of hemorrhagic strokes:

- **Intracerebral hemorrhage** is the most common type of hemorrhagic stroke. It occurs when an artery in the brain bursts, flooding the surrounding tissue with blood.

- **Subarachnoid hemorrhage** is a less common type of hemorrhagic stroke. It refers to bleeding in the area between the brain and the thin tissues that cover it.

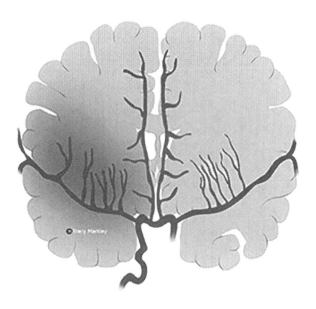

Transient Ischemic Attack (TIA)

A transient ischemic attack (TIA) is sometimes called a "mini-stroke." It is different from the major types of stroke because blood flow to the brain is blocked for only a short time, usually no more than five minutes. It can be from a few seconds up to five minutes. Your blood delivers oxygen to every part of your body. Your cells need it to survive. When blood flow gets blocked anywhere, it can be dangerous. TIAs are short and usually won't cause lasting damage, but it's still important to treat them like an emergency and get care right away. It is common that some TIAs are unnoticed and undiagnosed. Often, if this is the case, the patient's doctor can see in a scan that they have had one in the past.

It is important to know that:

- A TIA is a warning sign of a future stroke.

- A TIA is a medical emergency, just like a major stroke.

- Strokes and TIAs require emergency care. **Call 9-1-1** right away if you feel signs of a stroke or see symptoms in someone around you.

- There is no way to know in the beginning whether symptoms are from a TIA or from a major type of stroke.

- Like ischemic strokes, blood clots often cause TIAs.

- More than a third of people who have a TIA and don't get treatment have a major stroke within one year. As many as 10% to 15% of people will have a major stroke within three months of a TIA.

A stroke causes some brain cells to die and others to become injured. The injured cells are often found around the main area of damage. This area of injured cells is known as the penumbra. This is known as **Ischemic penumbra**. These cells may heal in the first few days and weeks after the stroke, which can cause some **spontaneous recovery.**

Cardio-embolic stroke A stroke due to a blood clot that has formed in the heart and travelled to the brain.

CHAPTER 3

BRAIN DAMAGE AND STROKE RECOVERY

As mentioned previously, adult brains make few or no neurons, therefore the biological damage is permanent. Strokes can cause serious motor and cognitive problems and sometimes permanent damage. Recovery depends on the remaining undamaged area of the brain. The after effect of a stroke is brain damage. The brain is like the software to the body, it malfunctions due to the stroke. The brain normally sends messages through the nerves to parts of the body to make movement through neuro pathways. After a stroke these messages hit road blocks

A simple way to describe this would be when the brain is trying to get a message to a specific part of the body to make a movement, the message cannot get through because the wires in the messaging system are not working properly. The brain now has to create new pathways, to get the message sent and received properly, as it did before the stroke. For example, if you were following directions on a road map to travel from point A to point B and you run into roadblocks, you have to figure out alternative routes to get to your destination. In many cases, the brain rebuilds these new pathways. We cannot predict which new pathways will appear, the time frame they will appear, nor the order in which they will appear. There is no time frame or limits on this process, especially if the body stays in motion as much as possible.

When the brain is trying to make new pathways and repair itself, it is called brain plasticity, or neuroplasticity. Neuroplasticity is the brain's ability to reorganize and rewire itself. It is trying to heal. The brain has an amazing ability to form new connections between brain cells. It has the ability to change throughout life.

The brain uses about 20% of the body's energy, but after a stroke, it uses much more of the body's energy due to the fact that it is trying to repair itself. The brain needs rest and sleep to heal. You may find many survivor's common complaint or concern is their constant fatigue or the need to sleep. This is usually normal. It is always important to know all their medical conditions and medications they are taking. Some brain injuries can cause insomnia as well.

When a survivor is recovering, they often will fatigue more quickly than they used to before their stroke. When a survivor is working with a therapist or a fitness professional for care, it is important to keep them aware of this and also share with the professional the survivor's daily activities, sleep and eating habits. Determining their exercise level and ability for each workout must be based on each individual session. Communication is essential. Finding a professional who will listen and understand this will help the survivor greatly. The more knowledge a fitness professional has about the anatomy, physiology and movement of the body, the better chance the professional can connect to the survivor's needs. The professional can adjust training sessions according to any changes in recovery the survivor's body has made.

With any client's goals in fitness, whether it's losing weight, getting stronger, training for an event or something such as stroke recovery, each client has to do their part every day, on their own, as well as in their time with a fitness professional. As we see with clients in weight loss that they have behaviors and mindsets that hold them back from results, professionals will find the same with stroke survivors.

As you continue through this book you will learn more about the many dynamics that play a role in stroke recovery.

There are many factors in play in recovery:

- Proper physical therapy
- Neurological exercises

- Staying consistent and repetitive in movements everyday
- A heathy diet
- Staying properly hydrated
- Mindset
- Support system
- Intensity of the brain damage from the stroke
- Time
- Patience
- Sleep and getting plenty of rest
- Other health conditions or injuries
- Motivation
- Emotional well being
- Sometimes age makes a difference
- Persistency
- Stress
- Other options a survivor is trying

If you don't know this yet, please know that stroke recovery is not an easy step-by-step process. I share with professionals that knowing as much as they can about the anatomy and biomechanics of the human body will help them as a fitness professional to guide the survivor into greater recovery.

The body was made to move. The more the body tries to move, the more chance the brain can rebuild its pathways for the movements. Survivors have a better chance of recovering if they do their exercises and walk every day, if they are able. Unfortunately, not all survivors understand this. Once they begin their outpatient therapy, they usually see the therapist once or twice a week. This is not enough. They need to continue, if possible, to work on their physical recovery daily with movement. Physical therapists and fitness professionals rarely get to train any client every day or almost every day of the week. I have only experienced this two times.

Although I have trained many survivors in the last 20 years, I had a special opportunity to train a 65-year-old gentleman who had a stroke six months prior to us meeting. We met when he walked into the gym in a walker. He trained with me five to six days a week for almost three years. This opportunity to see his changes in recovery in person on almost a daily basis, was not only incredible to witness the process, but extremely educational. It was also tremendous for his recovery. His journey was a perfect example of how the brain heals in no planned order. He was an example of a survivor who was connected to the awareness of the changes happening in his recovery, as well as what can happen when the trainer and survivor have good communication to help them work together as a team in survivor recovery.

Unfortunately, as I mentioned, it is rare that a survivor can meet with us daily. I find the more I can educate the survivor and their family and/or caregivers with them, (if they have them), the better chance they can try to push through. A survivor needs to move and exercise daily. In a way, it is as if they are training to become an athlete in their recovery. Athletes train for hours, almost daily. I know this is not possible for many survivors, but they need to move as much as possible in the movements they are trying to gain back.

Repetitive movement and consistency are essential. Proper nutrition and hydrating are also essential for brain care and health.

Due to the vast differences of damage and challenges each individual survivor is facing after their stroke, their starting point when they meet us as fitness professionals will all be different. Their limitations, energy levels and fatigue point will all be different. When a professional knows this, it will help the survivor get better care.

In my research of the brain, I listened to a neuroscientist discuss music therapy for the brain. In this lecture, he discussed music therapy in stroke survivors.

In this study they had survivors listen to an hour of self-selected music a day.

The study found that there were no changes soon after the stroke, but at three to six months post stroke, there were significant differences. In the cognitive tests, the verbal memory and focused attention were better than those who did not listen to an hour of self-selected music a day. The findings focused on mood measures showed those who listened to their music an hour a day showed signifyingly less depression than those who did not listen to music. They found that listening to this music enhanced cognition and mood after a stroke.

Those who listened to music did better on verbal memory, focused attention and may have felt less stressed.

Stress can also have a major effect on the brain. After someone has a stroke, it is normal if they feel major stress. Their body is not working, some may lose their job, their family, the ability to drive and other losses and challenges in their everyday life. If stress affects them to the point where the stress hormone enters the brain, it can affect the hippocampus, (learning and memory), frontal cortex (attention) and their amygdala (emotion regulation).

An MRI was also taken to look at the brain before and after the study. The brain study method used was *Voxel Based Morphometry or VBM*, to examine the changes in grey matter or white matter. They compared the first MRI performed right after they had their stroke to an MRI six months later. What they found was an increase of grey matter. An increase in grey matter helps sprouting of axons, branching of dendrites, formation of new synapses and an increase in small blood vessels in the brain. These changes are micro architectural of the brain. Those with left hemisphere strokes showed more grey matter in the superior frontal gyrus, which is cognitive processing. They also showed more grey matter in parts of the brain that is emotional processing. This showed that at six months post stroke they had structural reorganization in an adult brain of a stroke survivor. Although more studies are always being done, at the time of this study, they thought listening to music the first six months after a stroke may be the most critical time to use music therapy. They also recommend going to a certified music therapist when able.

I shared that study to help survivors, caregivers and professionals to understand why some survivors will exercise better and understand direction better when there is music playing or they listen to it often on their own, not even being aware of this study.

I shared that I had an 89-year-old survivor who would walk faster forward and back and more coordinated when I played music from his favorite CD. If I had him walk for 10 to 15 minutes with his favorite music playing before our exercise session where we worked on balance and the spasticity in his hand, he performed better and had a better workout. He was happier doing it as well. He had a memory challenge. He could not remember what he ate for lunch an hour before I saw him, but he could remember the band he played in 50 years prior. He also had a touch of dementia after his stroke and sometimes would lash out. Then he would forget he did it.

I had another survivor in his 60s who would stand on the BOSU® ball for 10 to 15 minutes listening to his favorite music before I even got to the gym in the mornings. I was not aware of this study at the time I was working with both of these survivors, although I was aware of the positive difference it made in the workout and progress.

CHAPTER 4

EVERY STROKE SURVIVOR WILL BE DIFFERENT

When I asked several stroke survivors about what challenges they faced while trying to find good guidance in recovery, many said "They treat us all the same. They need to understand that not all stroke survivors are the same."

Common impairments for stroke survivors are balance, memory, spasticity, numbness, limitation of movement and/or paralyzed on one side, speech, ability to read lost, hearing, foot drop/drag and aphasia. Some have a new outlook on life and are grateful to be alive while others may be in a state of depression and/or very upset they had a stroke. They often are angry at their own body. I actually had two different male stroke survivors, who speak English, tell me when they became alert and first spoke at the hospital after their strokes, they spoke in Spanish. One of them told me he never spoke Spanish in his life, but as his memory continued to return, he remembered that he was in the military years prior and had to speak Spanish on occasion.

I have found that what the survivor did for therapy before they were released on their own can vary greatly. Some have had the best therapy, and some have encountered not so good. What they experience in therapy, as care and results, can leave a survivor extremely discouraged or motivated. When I asked groups of survivors what they wish we knew or did in our work with them as fitness professionals, most of them said they wished professionals, being trainers or therapists, would explain to them why they are doing a specific exercise. I find with every client, if they understand why they are doing a movement or exercise, it helps them become aware of their body better. It helps them relate the exercise to a movement in everyday life they are trying to get back. If they understand a particular exercise will help build the body to do a movement needed for an activity, like riding their bike again, driving a car or picking up a child or grandchild safely as examples, it gives them hope and motivation. This gives them a goal and something to push for.

The fatigue and energy levels will vary person to person. It will also vary individually day to day. As professionals, we meet survivors from weeks to years post stroke. It will depend on the level of their stroke, damage, therapy and life occurrences. Whatever a survivor had going on physically before their stroke is still there. For example: Here is the condition of one of the survivors I trained five to six days a week when we met.

Six-month post stroke 65-year-old male.

Using a walker and sometimes a cane.

Knee surgery two weeks prior to his stroke. This left him with a weak hyper-extended knee, that never had physical therapy. Strokes can also cause hyperextended knees.

A rotator cuff injury on the same side the stroke affected.

Poor posture with Forward Head Posture (A condition where the position of the head moves forward from the center of the shoulders).

He had never stepped foot into a gym or worked out, except being a surfer in his younger years.

Numbness, spasticity and loss of sensations throughout the right side.

A brace on his right lower leg.

Foot drop and turn out on the right side.

Memory loss. It took him a couple months to remember my name. He always remembered me, but the name was a challenge to his memory.

Lost the ability to read, write and do his artwork.

Peripheral vision loss on the right.

Loss of Cutaneous Sensation in right hand - (Touch and everything else we feel through our skin such as temperature, texture, pressure, vibration and pain). These receptors also let the body know when things are hot or cold.

In the middle of a sentence a word was hard to find and speak.

Very little core stabilization.

Loss of spatial awareness and "Feeling safe" in everyday movements, like walking.

He did have a huge positive outlook and he was the most determined person I ever met to get better. He also had another important thing going for him. He told me he trusted me during our second meeting. If the survivor feels safe and trusts the fitness professional helping them, they will continue to come and do what is needed to get well.

As with all clients, when we make that kind of connection, the outcome can be better. As a fitness professional, we don't always have control of making this sort of connection. The client plays an important role in it, no matter how much we are there, some clients don't connect. Often, I find these clients may not be making a connection within themselves.

Besides the variety of challenges each survivor has, how in tune they are with themselves can make a big difference in recovery. When they understand why they are doing specific exercises and the muscles they are working, it forces them to make a connection to their body. Often survivors are left to rely on their family and caregivers to communicate for them. This leaves whoever is helping them to be their communicator to any professional trying to help. In these cases, I do my bet to educate the caregivers and helpers.

When they can connect to even the smallest changes coming back in recovery, it helps us as professionals know where they are at each time we train them. It is a good signal and direction from their brain telling them changes are taking place. For Example: A particular survivor client used to tell me in the beginning of workout sessions, "I know this doesn't mean much but look what I can do." He may show me that he can kneel on one leg and get up without holding on. It could have been he showed me that he can open his hand a bit further then the last training session or tell me he can move and feel his pinky finger now. Whatever he expressed, he would think it is no big deal, but he knew I wanted to know everything. As professionals, if we understand the mechanics of the body, this sort of communicating tells us what their body is doing. As for kneeling on one leg on the floor and getting up now, it just told me that his core, knee, pelvic, hamstrings, glutes and ankle stabilization are getting stronger and that he is feeling safer in movements. This showed me his body is on its way to gaining back some daily activities like washing a car, getting clothes out of a dryer, yard work and getting things out of and putting things into cupboards. His motivation, confidence and hope has built higher as well.

As for the feeling and movement coming back into the pinky finger, this tells me a few things. One, that the posture of his head and neck has improved. His gripping and holding objects will improve. The neck, elbow, wrist, hand and fingers will most likely begin to see more changes and strength building. He then could begin raising the amount of weight for biceps and triceps as well as do more variations of exercises for the upper back, shoulders and arms. The nerves to the hands and fingers come from the neck. The Laser Spine Institute explains the ulna nerve very nicely.

"The ulna nerve roots are where the nerves branch off the spinal cord between C7 and T1 vertebrae. This nerve's root helps facilitate the flow of signals between the brain and the arms. To accomplish this, the brain sends messages down the spinal cord, through the nerve root then along the ulnar nerve and back again almost instantaneously. Specifically, the ulnar nerve extends from the spinal cord through the arm, forearm, hand and into the little finger. But what makes the ulnar nerve unique is that it is the largest nerve in the body that has an unprotected spot, known as the funny bone."

Another Example: An 82-year-old survivor has aphasia. His 82-year-old wife shared with me one day that when he was sleeping, his leg twitched, which is normal, but this particular night after we did some exercises with the legs, she said there was more twitching and more activity going on. This was a good thing. This was an excellent report back to me. I now knew how the work he was doing was changing the body. The more a survivor and/or their caregivers can be aware of things they see, even if they sound silly, the better the professional can help, especially if the professional has the knowledge to work with it.

The more awareness we have of a survivor's changes, the better for them as well. They may not notice changes like we can. Another example, when a male survivor walked up to a chair and sat down normally. I asked him if he noticed what he just did. He said, "No. What?" I shared with him that he used to walk slowly to a chair, turned around very slowly to sit down at the front of the chair as he held on to the chair and slowly slid himself back in the seat. Which is very common when one loses the awareness of where their feet are in space. There is a re-enactment of this on my YouTube channel. (Tracy L. Markley Fitness). This means he can step backwards safety and he had re-gained subconsciously the steps of his feet. (More about this in the Spatial Awareness chapter and the Walking chapter).

CHAPTER 5

COMMUNICATION IS CRUCIAL

In the last chapter, I shared some examples of how communicating to the professional is very helpful for the survivor and the professional. It is crucial to have clear communication between my client and me. I regularly ask clients questions to be sure they are feeling the specific exercise where the exercise was intended to be felt. When I asked the group of survivors what challenges they faced when trying to find help to further their recovery, the most popular answers were "They don't listen." and "They treat us as irrelevant."

I know reading my words in this book where I tell survivors and their caregivers to find a professional who listens may sound like an easy task, but it may not be. This is important. I find at times clients may appear to be doing an exercise correctly, but may be feeling it in a different place than I planned for various reasons. They may need to correct their form, but they can't. I need to know if it is because the client does not understand or their body cannot physically do what I am asking. For example: A client is feeling their neck while doing a bicep curl because he is tensing his neck and shoulders internally but not enough for me to see his shoulders raise up, or when a client is in perfect form for a squat, but their knee begins to hurt. In order for me to serve the clients the best I can, these things are necessary for me to know. I also need to know how hard or easy an exercise is for them.

When a client has numbness throughout their body and their brain cannot connect to what the body is doing or feeling, it can make the communication a bigger challenge. A survivor may not understand what it means to "feel fatigue" in a muscle from working out. This is when most of us know our limit. There is a difference between muscle fatigue and a muscle that is numb and not getting all the messages from the brain to perform at its best. If a survivor has never exercised or experienced the feeling and sense of exercise fatigue, this can be like a foreign language.

These situations are when professionals need to be aware and play the role as the client's second brain to help them stay safe. I ask questions repeatedly to make sure they don't get up from a machine or the ball and collapse to the floor because the stroke-affected leg gave out. It is often difficult for survivors to know and then explain what they were feeling or not feeling. A survivor may feel bad sometimes because they cannot communicate what they want to say. At times, the brain won't process a word they want to say as quickly as it did before their stroke. It can be exhausting for the survivor. As a professional or caregiver, always be patient and kind when a survivor is trying to communicate to you. It often will take longer than someone who has not had a stroke. This will make them feel better communicating with you as well as giving them a sense to be okay with where they are in their communicating skills. Never make them feel like they are stupid or unimportant. When I asked the stroke survivor groups what they would like changed by professionals, as I shared earlier, a big issue expressed was that they were treated as if they were irrelevant. No one wants to feel irrelevant.

A survivor may have aphasia. Aphasia is a communication disorder that impairs a person's ability to process language. It does not affect intelligence. Aphasia impairs the ability to speak and understand others. It can affect the ability to read and write. There is also non-fluent aphasia. This is when a person cannot talk or get words out, but they can sing a song or a sentence.

I have been working with a stroke survivor client who can say one word randomly, but he can sing songs and sing full sentences with no problem. I have been trying to encourage him and his wife to communicate in singing. It would be great for his brain and learning to talk again. It could also help a hard situation be possibly fun and bring them laughter. Laughter is always healing.

As a part of communicating with a client, we also have to determine the balance of their exercises they are doing at home with each workout they attend with us. Like everyone, survivor's need to keep moving daily, but not overdo it. They also need proper recovery. Finding that balance when a client cannot feel all the sensations in their body, is quite difficult.

A cell phone is a great tool for communicating with a client in person. Since many survivors do not like looking at themselves in a mirror, especially when they are trying to exercise. I found taking a picture or video to show them has been an excellent source in communication. One example is when a client is working on their foot drop and turn out while walking. I would video the client's feet from the front of the treadmill or them walking down the hall, so they can see what needed to be changed or what had changed. Some survivors, if possible, who have a treadmill at home put a mirror in front of the treadmill to watch their legs and feet while walking on the treadmill. Here is another example with one of my male survivors; as he progressed, he was able to perform a plank exercise. A survivor may not always understand verbal directions to get into proper form. If a client can see a picture of themself doing a particular exercise and me doing the same exercise, they can then see more clearly the directions I was giving. This process of communication is fabulous, not only for the communication aspect, but I can use the pictures later on in a survivor's journey, so they can see just how far they have progressed from earlier times. I have used this to help clients see their progress in their posture gains and other gains. They get excited to see how far they have come. They don't always understand or see the depth of progress achieved. This makes them feel great and inspires them to keep pushing forward and to never give up.

One reason looking in the mirror is hard for some survivors is that their perception of where they are in space is off. If they try to watch themselves exercise in the mirror to check for proper form, it may not be easy for them. If they have a loss of peripheral vision on one side, that can make it more complicated. The message to the brain sent for movement is struggling. If they try to watch themselves in the mirror and make the movements, it may complicate things even more. Sometimes it is best to keep them staying focused on the movement they are trying to achieve. Some survivor clients still do not look at themselves in the mirror, this is very common. When I was training a 65-year-old stroke survivor one day, he told me that he did not understand why. I explained to him that he spent 65 years knowing who he was when he looked at himself, but after the stroke, he saw himself differently. I shared with him that there was a time in my life when I was very ill for a few years, and when I looked in the mirror, I did not see me. I saw a stranger, and I felt like a stranger, in my own body. He responded with, "Exactly!" When one has a stroke, they feel like they are a stranger to their own body.

If a client feels frustrated or down because they are not making progress, I take out my phone and show the client the videos and pictures of the progress they have achieved. This is powerful. They literally can see the changes that they sometimes don't connect or notice. They are looking for big changes most of the time and don't always understand how important the changes are they have achieved. The cell phone can be an excellent tool for motivation.

National Aphasia Association. www.aphasia.org is a good source for aphasia.

Check out "The Stroke of An Artist, The Journey of a Fitness Trainer and A Stroke Survivor," by Tracy L. Markley.

CHAPTER 6

REBUILDING THE BODY – BIOMECHANICS AND MUSCLES

This may be the longest and most complex chapter in the book. I try to teach other professionals that having a greater knowledge of the mechanics of the human body and movement will help them bring survivors to greater recovery. The more the survivor and caregivers understand, it will help recovery too. In this chapter, I will go over some of the important muscles for stabilizing and movement of the body. As you look at the muscle illustrations, you will gain a better understanding of how important it is to have the center of the body strong and stable.

Stroke survivors, as well as all of us, need these muscles to be strong and working together as a team for proper movement. That will help achieve a balanced body and walking gait that will lead to being safer in movement.

Scientific research has shown that in a healthy body, the brain sends a message to specific muscles in the core of the body, before it sends a message to the legs and the arms for movement. This is called centrally generated motor pattern and means we recruit from the core outwards for movement of the body. This is the brain communicating to these muscles to stabilize and support the body, because it is ready to move. I like to call this the balancing system of the body. With this in mind, for example, if a client has had a stroke, the brain is already having a hard time getting messages throughout the body for proper movement. The brain is trying to create new pathways of communication because the old pathways are not working properly. It makes sense to me, that if the stabilizing muscles are weak and not functioning to their full potential, it could cause the rebuilding of pathways to the limbs to be more difficult to achieve.

When the core of the body is strong, it will stabilize the body mechanically as it is meant to do. The limbs then can become stronger and work in better movement with the body as a team, like it is meant to do. The core links the upper body and the lower body in movements.

There is less stress on the body physiologically when the biomechanics are functioning properly. Physiology focuses on the systems and organs of the body and their functions. Holding your body upright in a proper posture, not only looks better and helps the body to balance better, it makes the systems in the body work and function better. It helps the communication from the brain to the limbs to flow more naturally.

It is also important to understand that each muscle in the body has a specific job to do in moving the body. If some muscles are too weak to perform the job they were meant to do, other muscles try to do the job for them. This is like a sports team with players that can't play the sport very well, it throws the whole team off.

Anatomy

The **transverse abdominal muscle**, the **multifidus muscle**, **diaphragm** and the **pelvic floor muscles** are all on the same neuromuscular loop. This means it is best if all these muscles are functioning properly; each needs to perform its job individually <u>and</u> as a team. If the transverse muscle is weak, the pelvic floor, the multifidus and the diaphragm cannot gain proper strength to perform their jobs in a healthy, functioning body.

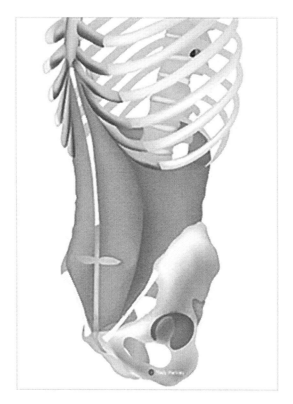

The **transverse muscle** is the deepest of the abdominal muscles. A critical function of this muscle is to stabilize the lower back and pelvis before movement. It is the deepest abdominal muscle, wrapping around the body to act like a corset. When engaged, it also pulls the belly in and provides support to the **thoracolumbar fascia**, and it is the stabilizer of the shoulder girdle, the head, neck, pelvis and lower extremities.

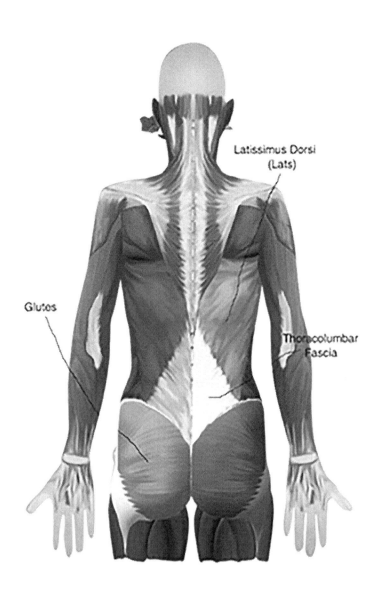

If a client has rounded shoulders and poor posture, it will not be corrected if the transverse muscle maintains the weakness. The transverse muscle needs to be strengthened, along with the other stabilizing muscles, to hold the body strongly upright, so that it can achieve a posture in which the shoulders are stacked over the hips. If the head is upright and balanced over the shoulders, we have better balance. Survivors need to rebuild stability in the pelvis and hips, so that the lower limbs and joints can gain strength, function in alignment and perform properly for safe movements.

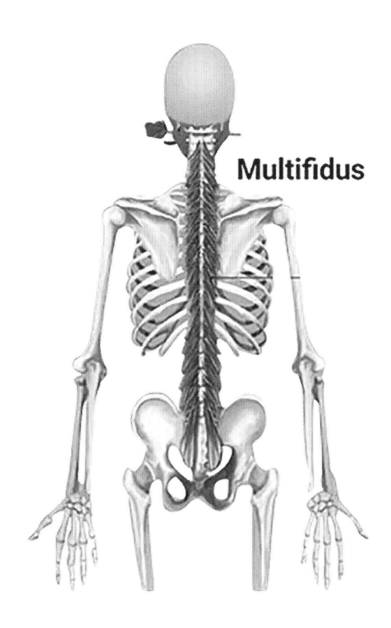

Multifidus

The **multifidus** is a small but powerful muscle. It is the main stabilizing muscle of the spine. This muscle takes pressure off the vertebral discs, so that the body weight can be distributed throughout the spine. If this is weak, you will also have weakness in the low back. The **multifidus** begins to activate before the body moves to protect the spine. It is part of the stabilizing system in the body. In order to gain better balance, this muscle must be stronger. Performing various exercises combining with the Swiss ball, balance disc and BOSU® ball will help gain a stronger multifidus. Better posture leads to better balance.

The small muscles near the vertebrae need to be activated harmoniously. These muscles are postural muscles. Exercising on an unstable surface, such as the Swiss ball, balance disc and the BOSU® ball, stimulates the central nervous system, which is the brain and the spinal cord. It strengthens muscles and ligaments, as well as activating and strengthening all the small muscles along the spinal column.

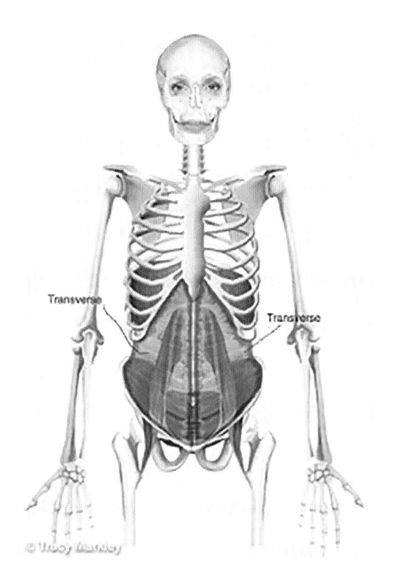

The **pelvic floor** muscles work as stabilizers of
the abdominal and pelvic organs. The pelvic floor

muscles and the gluteus (buttock) muscles are made to work and move in opposite directions. One must be able to engage the pelvic floor without engaging the gluteus muscles in order to obtain optimal core strength. These two muscles must be separated in the brain and nervous system for overall whole-body functioning. This plays a role in preventing back issues, and I don't want to build back issues in any client. The transverse muscle must be strong in order for the pelvic floor to become strong and function properly, since they are on the same neuromuscular loop.

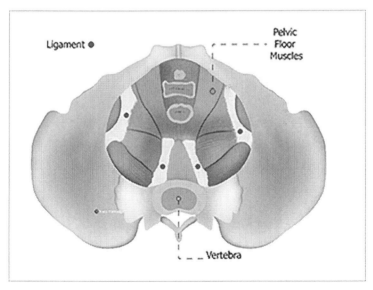

For the best results, I have the survivor engage the pelvic floor then visualize and feel that they are zipping up a zipper from the pelvic floor to their rib cage or sternum. The more conscious and present a client is when doing this, the better the chance, subconsciously, of these muscles contracting in everyday movements when needed, without thinking about it. It is important to remember to keep this focus throughout the exercises.

The **pelvic floor** works close to the diaphragm as well. If you sit or stand in good alignment and focus on engaging the pelvic floor, you can feel that the diaphragm pulls slightly towards the pelvic floor as the pelvic floor lifts slightly towards the diaphragm. There is a difference between doing a Kegel and engaging the pelvic floor. It is also important to be able to engage the pelvic floor without engaging the buttocks (glutes) for the inner unit and stabilizing system in the body to work efficiently.

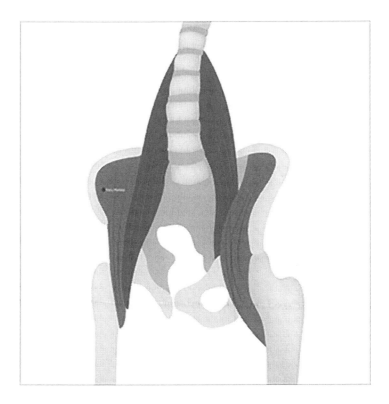

The **psoas muscle** is an extremely important muscle located in the center of the body. It lies deep underneath the transverse abdominal muscle. It is a deep back muscle. It is the bridge between the hips and the back. Often it is referred to as the iliopsoas. This is when the psoas and the iliacus muscles are being grouped together. The psoas muscle is the only muscle in the back that crosses over the hips and attaches at the front of the body. It attaches at the last thoracic vertebrae and to four of the five lumbar vertebrae and at the femur, the upper thigh bone. It is also the bridge between the hips and the back.

As Evan Osar explains in his book "The Psoas Solution," *The psoas has extensive fascial attachments to the trunk, spine, pelvis and hips. Additionally, it fascially attaches to several muscles within these regions, including the diaphragm, quadratus lumborum, transverse abdominal, pelvic floor and iliacus.*

If the abdominals are weak, the **psoas** tries to perform the work of the abdominal. If the psoas is short, weak and/or tight it will be difficult to hold the body in an upright position with the shoulders stacked over the hips.

The psoas works closely with the diaphragm. The diaphragm is the main muscle for breathing. The psoas is the main muscle for walking. The psoas attaches at the lumbar spine and the crura of the diaphragm attaches there as well. The crura (plural for crus), are two fibroelastic bands that come up from the lumbar vertebrae and inserts into the central tendon of the diaphragm. There is one on the left side and one on the right side. Together they perform a muscle contraction. A person has to walk and breathe at the same time. The psoas and the diaphragm must be strong for movement and walking.

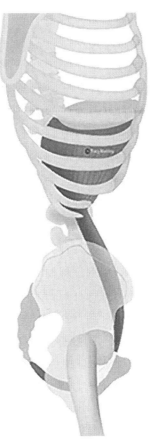

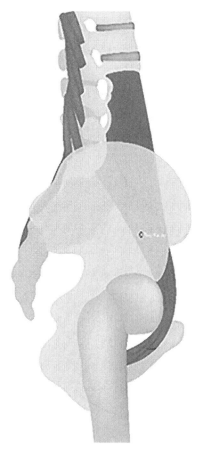

In the first illustration, you see a side view of the diaphragm and the psoas muscles. The second illustration is a partial side view of the multifidus and the psoas muscles.

To sum this chapter up, proper posture and sitting up tall does not begin at the shoulders. Let's strengthen from deep in the core to help straighten up. The center of the body must be strong to hold up the diaphragm, rib cage and shoulder girdles in proper alignment in order to have proper posture. The center of the body must be strong and balanced to keep the pelvic and hips stable and strong, which leads us to having a stronger, more balanced and safer walking gait.

Quadratus Lumborum

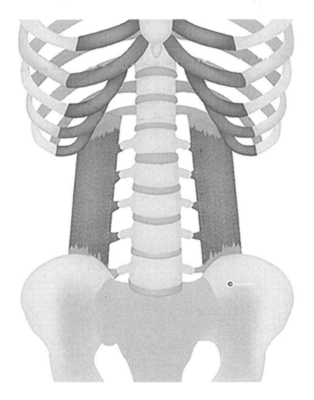

The quadratus lumborum (as you can see in illustration above) is attached from the lumbar vertebrae and rib 12 to the crest of the ilium. It stabilizes the pelvis (hip girdle), as in walking, and laterally flexes the spine. When this muscle is only activated (or in spasticity) on one side, the trunk is bent towards that direction.

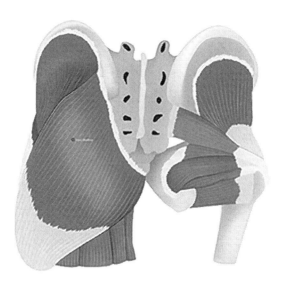

In this illustration, you will see the large glute muscles and the smaller muscles that are underneath. The large glute muscles extend the femur, which is the back swing of the leg in walking. It also rotates the femur outward. The smaller group of muscles work together to rotate the femur outward. The femur is the large upper thigh bone.

The Sciatica Nerve

As trainers and therapists, when we hear "sciatica nerve" we instantly think pain. Although the sciatica nerve is said to be the largest single nerve in the body, it is made up of five nerves. It is found on the right and left side of the lower spine by the fourth and fifth lumbar nerves and the first three nerves in the sacral spine. At the largest part of the nerve, it is as big as a male thumb. The five nerves group together on the front of the piriformis muscles and become one large nerve, known as the sciatic nerve. This nerve supplies sensation and strength to the leg and the reflexes of the leg. It connects the spinal cord with the outside of the thigh, the hamstring muscles and the muscles of the lower leg and feet. It provides motor and sensory functions to regions of the leg and foot. When the sciatic nerve is impaired, it can lead to muscle weakness and/or numbness and tingling in the leg, ankle, foot and toes. The sciatic nerve and its nerve branches enable movement and feeling in the thigh, knee, calf, ankle, foot and toes.

With this in mind, you can better visualize the importance of strengthening and balancing the deep core and spinal muscles as well as stimulating the central nervous system.

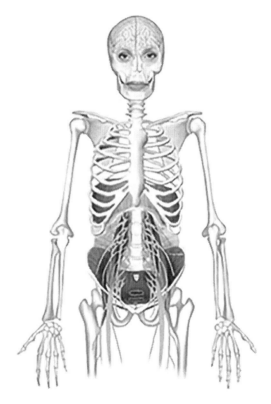

In this illustration, I show just some of the nerves going through the core of the body. I share this illustration to help give a "visual" and "understanding" of the importance of core strength and proper posture.

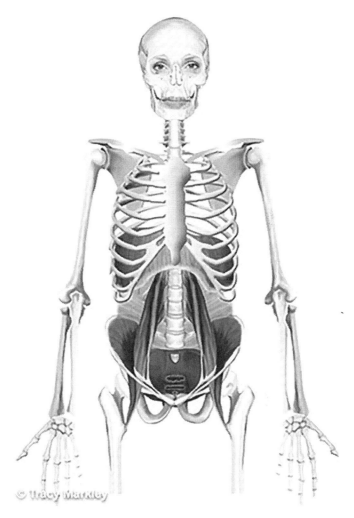

I share this illustration to help give a "visual" and "understanding" of the importance of core strength and proper posture.

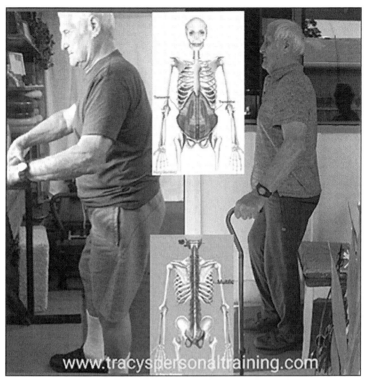

The center of the body must be strong to hold the body upright in proper alignment. In the above photo is an 82-year-old stroke survivor. He was almost four years post stroke when I met him. This is one week of work together. If a client has a drop foot, if the muscles in the center of the body becomes stronger, the leg and foot may begin to re-establish proper stepping. A survivor will have better recovery in their walking gait, if they combine a strong posture with their physical therapy exercises for drop foot.

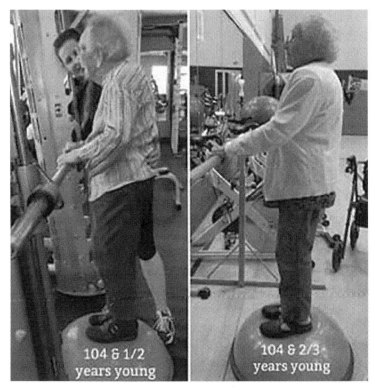

In this photo you can see her posture changed in just 3 months. She was 104 years old.

CHAPTER 7

BRAIN CARE

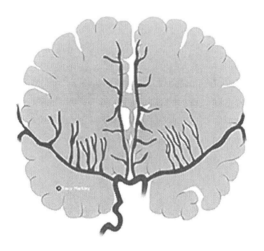

The brain is one of the largest and most complex organs in your body. It is made up of more than 100 billion nerves that communicate in trillions of connections called synapses. It is very active metabolically. It receives 20% of the cardio output. The brain has very little or no ability to store oxygen or glucose. Neurons die within minutes if deprived of oxygen. Anything that cuts off blood flow to the brain compromises brain function. Neurons die and they are not replaced.

The brain uses 20% of the body's energy in a healthy body. When the brain is trying to recover from a stroke and brain damage, it uses much more energy. This leaves survivors feeling fatigued. This is normal. It is important that they get the rest needed and understand that fatigue is what happens in the process of the brain trying to heal itself.

It is important to take good care of neurons that take care of the vessels that supply oxygen to the brain. The entire blood supply to the brain is from two major arterial systems: The internal carotid and the vertebral systems. The internal is part of the circulation, primarily to the front of the brain. Vertebral arteries supply the brain stem and cerebellum. In a healthy brain, the muscles move on commands from the brain. There are single nerve cells in the spinal cord, called motor neurons, and they are the way the brain connects to muscles.

The brain is 80% water. The body is 75% water. The bones are 25% water. It is essential for us to drink water and stay hydrated. Many people go about their everyday life maintaining a stage of dehydration. When one combines a dehydrated brain, poor nutrition and lack of exercise, it will definitely encourage the aging process in all our organs, including the brain. When a brain with an injury maintains a stage of dehydration it can impair the healing process.

Your brain needs water! It provides a fluid balance for all chemical reactions in the body. It is a lubricant and plays a vital role in regulating your body temperature. Water flushes out toxins and waste from our organs. Your brain is an organ. The brain is one of the largest and most complex organs in your body. Your skin is the largest organ in the body, and staying hydrated can create clearer skin and can help with anti-aging of the skin. In a dehydrated brain, the very complex functions of the brain get disorganized and makes the whole body have issues. Even a mildly or temporarily dehydrated brain can alter brain function. Even in the adult brain, neurons continue to form new connections and strengthen existing connections

If the brain is dehydrated or even slightly dehydrated, it can lead to feeling brain fog, sluggish, tired, irritable and more. It can even affect one's memory. It also can slow down the process of the brain making neurons and other highly important functions the body needs as well as keeping the brain healthy and fit and able to function at its best.

Research has also shown that the brain volume peaks at age 40, then begins to decline 5% every 10 years. We must do everything possible to fight against this process by not adding to that percentage with poor hydration. A dehydrated brain shrinks in volume, slows down the metabolism and can increase cholesterol level.

Brain Specific Exercises stimulate the central nervous system. Scientific studies also show that aerobic exercise stimulates the hypothalamus.

Resources: "Your Brain: The Software to Your Body, A Fitness Trainer's Guide to Brain Health," by Tracy L. Markley

The Great Courses on the Brain "Tipping Toward Balance: A Fitness Trainer's Guide to Stability and Balance," by Tracy L. Markley

CHAPTER 8

FASCIA

Fascia is a continuous structure that surrounds and intermingles tissues and structures throughout the body. It varies in density and thickness. Nerves and blood vessels also run through fascia. When the brain is sending messages for movement, it includes the fascia. Training survivors with knowledge of fascia is important, while choosing which exercises are the best for each client. Fascia is also interconnected with the structures it surrounds. The health and mobility of fascia plays a huge role for the body to have heathy movement, and to avoid pain and injury. There are ongoing studies on fascia and its mandatory importance for the body to move.

"Fascia contains mechanoreceptors and proprioceptors. In other words, every time we use a muscle, we stretch fascia that is connected to spindle cells, Ruffini and Paccini corpuscles and Golgi organs. The normal stretching of fascia thus communicates the force of the muscle contraction and the status of the muscle regarding its tone, movement, rate of change in muscle length and position of the associated body part to the central nervous system." **From Dr. Warren Hammer, the chiropractic profession's leading expert in soft tissues and fascia ("The Fascial System is a Sensory Organ").**

Dr. Hammer went on to say in another article ("Why We Need to Fix the Mechanoreceptors"*)*

that, *"One of the most relevant discoveries in the world of anatomy over these many years is that muscle spindles, the chief proprioceptive cells affecting our muscles, are not in the muscle, but in the fascia surrounding the muscle and its muscle bundles. A mechanoreceptor is stimulated when it is deformed, but when it is restricted in fascia that is unable to glide... it is unable to stretch, which is critical for the function of the spindle cell."*

The thoracolumbar fascia is an important fascia to understand. It is necessary for walking, running and mobility. When a professional has the knowledge of the fascia and exercising through the fascia lines, it gives them more avenues to help survivors gain back movement. This sort of knowledge can be an excellent addition in training a stroke survivor and helping their brain make new pathways for the movements needed.

Thoracolumbar Fascia

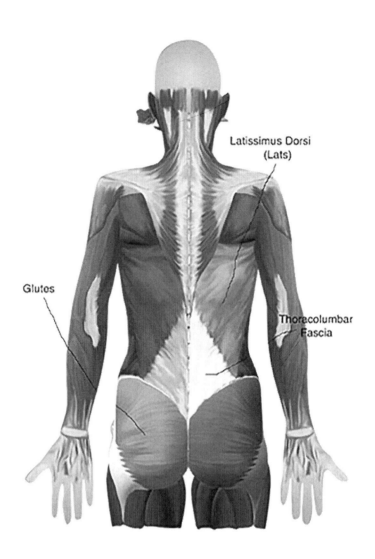

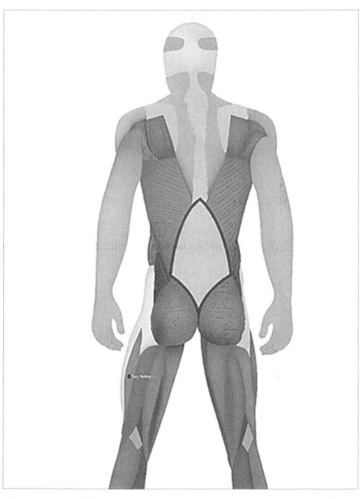

The above illustration is to give another visual of the thoracolumbar fascia.

The thoracolumbar fascia supports the back muscles and helps them achieve the ability to move the body. It is made up of strong fibers and helps channel forces of movement, as the back muscles contract and relax. The nerves to these muscles also cross through this fascia. This fascia goes deep to the spine and is made of three layers. It is essential for contralateral motions like walking. It works with the latissimus dorsi (lats) to coil the core of the body.

When the thoracolumbar fascia is supported, it allows all the muscles that connect to it function better. These muscles include the gluteus maximus, latissimus dorsi, trapezius, erector spine, quadratus lumborum, psoas, transverse and internal obliques. It helps bridge the muscles of the back to the muscles of the abdominal wall. This fascia helps integrate the movements of the upper body with the lower body.

We also have a posterior **Oblique Subsystem** (which is not the exact opposite of the oblique abdominal muscles despite the similar name). This system consists of:

- Latissimus Dorsi Muscle

- Thoracolumbar Fascia (not a muscle)

- Contralateral Gluteus Maximus Muscle (some also consider the Gluteus Medius a part as well).

Chapter 9

Treadmill and Walking

B y the time a survivor has met their fitness professional, they may have been already walking slowly on the treadmill in therapy and/or at home. It's not unusual if they have not been doing this. If they are able, get them walking on a treadmill, holding on safely to help get the locomotion for walking going. A study from the Cleveland Clinic stated that walking was one of the best things to do after a stroke. It stated that the soonest a survivor can try to get the body to perform locomotion, as in walking, the sooner the walking gait can come back.

One of the things to have a client focus on while on the the treadmill is to be present and conscious and to keep the stroke-affected foot pointing forward as much as possible. This requires being focused every second on their foot placement when they walk. If a client just walks on the treadmill and watches television and/or is not paying attention to their posture, form and stepping, they will not gain the progress needed or possible.

An important impact of the walking gait is stabilization and strength of the pelvic girdle, which leads us right back to the core and the deep stabilizing muscles of the body. When all that is stable, the lower limbs will be more stable, and can build their strength for functional movement at its best while avoiding injury.

If the client is able to walk on the treadmill without you monitoring them, it is a good place for them to warm up, even if it is walking very slowly. I like to have my clients come early, if they are able, and walk on the treadmill on their own time, so we have the full session to focus on all the other exercises needed for their case. If they are unable to walk safely without your supervision, please stay with them for their safety and guidance. There will be survivors who are not able to use the treadmill when you begin working with them. If a survivor has spasticity in one of their arms, they will not be able to hold onto the treadmill with both hands for safety. They may have spasticity in their leg that limits them from lifting up the leg safely enough to be using the treadmill. Help them gain strong core, balance and standing-up strength before trying to get them on a treadmill.

In the best survivor patient cases, the most fragile time in a survivor's recovery is spent with a physical therapist, before we begin working with them. This is not always the case.

Walking Backward and Backward Movements

Walking backward might seem silly, but it is good for you physically and mentally. We take steps backward often in our daily activity. Walking backward enhances the sense of body awareness. It increases body coordination and movement of the body in space. Research has shown walking backward improves the walking forward skills. It is said to sharpen your thinking skills, enhance cognitive control and put the senses into overdrive. This movement also puts less strain on and requires less range of motion from the knee joints.

◢It is very important for everyone to have awareness as to where the "body is in space." It is important for athletes to practice and train with focused awareness of where their body is in space for function, speed and agility. They gain better balance, speed and quicker reaction time, which are highly important skills for sports, especially fast-moving sports. Stroke survivors need to regain these skills for everyday life movements and regain quick reactions. Some examples: if they drive, moving quickly to the brake pedal when needed; moving their foot quickly to avoid tripping and falling or to avoid dropping an object on the floor.

One of my stroke survivors used to take big, wide circles of steps in order to turn around. I remember the day this particular survivor turned around normally. He lit up and said, "Did you see that?" I excitedly said, "Yes I did. That is so cool!"

I read studies that suggest having a client walk backward on a treadmill will help increase awareness and foot placement, but I am not comfortable with that. I feel walking backward on a treadmill belt can be unsafe for most clients. I suggest having any survivor do it on the floor in front of a mirror so they can see and feel their foot placement. If they don't like looking in the mirror, have them focus and watch just their feet and walking gait in the mirror.

I feel strongly that survivors in such fragile states must have their core stabilizing muscles before attempting to walk backward. Stability and safety are essential.

The following photos are of a client within two years of recovery. The first picture was the first month post stroke as he was still in the re-hab hospital. There were three physical therapists working with him. One pulled the machine, one was pushing it and the other was making his legs walk as he hung in the harness. Doctors did not think he was going to live the first two weeks. Every man in his family who had a stroke had died too. He beat those odds, and after two weeks, he was able to start some re-hab. I met him six months post stroke, and he was still in a walker. He was told he would be in a wheelchair the rest of his life. He was consistent in our work together and this second picture is over two years post stroke, and he was doing the running man on the BOSU® ball.

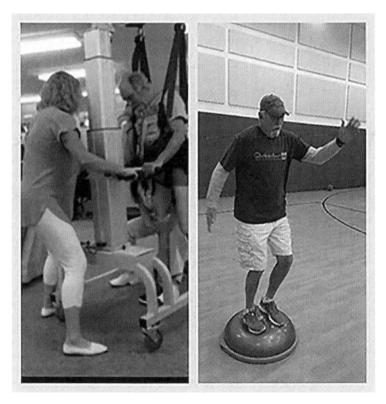

The pictures below are him a few months into rehab at the hospital he was still in. The picture with him walking with the cane is a couple months into our training together. The last picture of him walking and squatting on the BOSU® ball was taken about two and one-half years post stroke. His full recovery journey of us working together is now a book; "The Stroke of An Artist; The Journey of a Fitness Trainer and a Stroke Survivor." He wanted his journey shared to help teach professionals and to help other stroke survivors. I was happy to write the book.

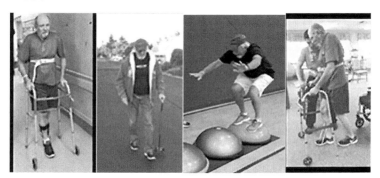

CHAPTER 10

FOCUS AND VISUALIZATION

When a survivor is trying to obtain a particular movement, such as lifting a foot or opening up a hand that has spasticity, it helps to have them focus and visualize what they are trying to achieve. For example: I will have a survivor focus on the hand that has not been affected by the stroke. I have them watch it open and close and hold the fingers out extended as far as they can. I ask them to see it, feel it, then close their eyes and stay with the vision and feeling of it performed properly. Then I will have them close their eyes and visualize the stroke affected hand doing the same thing. I have them try to see it and feel it, and often this will cause movement. If I have them stand on a balance disc and do the same thing, the movement will be bigger. In time the achieved opening of the hand will begin to remain open. This takes practicing daily, if possible, and as much as possible. Focus is very important. If they are standing on a balance disc, where the central nervous system is being stimulated, it can speed up the recovery progress.

Mirror Neurons: The existence of mirror neurons means you can gain skills through observation. Mirror neurons are involved in imitative learning through interactions with neural motor areas in humans. The application of mirror therapy techniques in post-stroke patients has demonstrated good results, especially when combined with other techniques. I find it works better with focus and visualization; and it works even better when a survivor can use the balance disc and BOSU® ball. Use a balance pad to stand on if the disc and BOSU® ball are not a task they can do yet.

Athletes often attribute their exceptional abilities to being able to "see" the ball and its flight prior to striking or catching it. The brain's ability to learn in this way makes a biological case for the use of simulations and case studies as tools in your quest for development as a leader. Such approaches not only promise effective ways of learning but are also potentially very efficient.

CHAPTER 11

SPATIAL AWARENESS, PROPRIOCEPTION AND FEELING SAFE IN MOVEMENTS

Spatial awareness is the ability to be conscious of oneself in space. It's to be mindful of where your body is and how much room you have around it and knowledge of the distance of objects in your surroundings. It is also referred to as proprioception—the placement of the body in relation to the things around it. It is the discernment of organized knowledge of the objects around oneself, in relation to the given space at any time, either still or when there is a change of position. It is relating to the height and depth of the objects around you, such as having to step over something on the floor when you are walking through a room. You must be able to relate to the height of the object you need to step over, so your foot lifts high enough and steps far enough out before landing back on the floor to clear the object. Spatial awareness is a complex cognitive skill. We learn this skill as children. It must be relearned in many cases after a stroke, as is the case with many stroke survivors.

Proprioception is sensing and knowing where the limbs are in space. Without adequate proprioception from the trunk and legs, it is difficult simply to walk into a room and sit down in a chair. Example: When you enter a room and are aware of how far to walk to the chair, the brain calculates the distance and the feet walk accordingly. The body starts taking smaller steps when needed, as well as adjusting the speed of each step as it approaches the chair to turn around. Now the brain calculates the turn and the size of steps and the direction of the steps required to place the body in the right position to prepare to sit. It then calculates the distance, height and where the seat of the chair is in space, as it coordinates with where the body is in space before it lowers the body to sit down safely. The brain directs the body, so it knows where it is in space to guide it down into sitting position in the chair without missing the chair and falling to the floor.

After a stroke, it can be difficult for a survivor to decipher verbal directions such as forward, back, right or left. This is called **confused positional languages**. This can be very common after a severe stroke. This makes it hard for a stroke victim to follow directions if they cannot see or follow something they can see. If a survivor also has proprioception and/or spatial awareness challenges, it will usually take them a bit longer to catch on to a movement or exercise. Don't give up on them. Be patient and understanding. Remember they are trying to be patient and understanding of their new strange body that won't do what they want it to do.

One day out of the blue, I had a client stop in the middle of a workout and explain to me that he knew there was the road with cars driving on it outside the gym and that there were people around him at the gym, but only because he knew it, not because he "saw" or "felt" them around him. The sense of his surroundings was not there. He was actually describing his loss of spatial awareness. I had not explained to him what that was, he just knew something was not normal in how he felt in his surroundings.

I remember the day this client began getting back his spatial awareness. He was at 18 months post stroke. He was standing on the balance disc when he stepped off the disc and said, "Wait, I need to share something." He made a small movement with his arms close to his body as if he were making a small circle around himself with his hands and said, "It's like my world used to stop here." Then he reached his arms and hands out as far as he could making a large circle around his body then said, "But now it ends here."

I felt such joy for him. It was fascinating. It felt magical the way he explained it. I said to myself, "Wow, he just got his awareness back. We just experienced him getting his awareness back. This is phenomenal!" Then I thought, "Oh my God, I helped him achieve that." I was joyfully overwhelmed in a "Wow" moment that lasted for days. It was beyond having a feeling of absolute fulfillment in my work. It remains one of my favorite moments with any client in my fitness career.

Proprioception

The word "proprioception" comes from two words. First is the Latin word *proprius*, meaning "one's own." The word "perception," meaning the process by which one translates sensory input into a coherent and unified picture of one's environment. Proprioception is the sense or "perception" of the relative position of various parts of the body in relationship to its environment. It is knowing where those various body parts are in space as well as how they are moving in relationship to each other. It is this internal sense, it tells you whether your body and limbs are moving, how fast they may be moving and how much energy is being expended to move a specific body part. It also tells us where various parts of the body are located in space in relation to every other part of the body. The brain integrates information from proprioception using all four brain hemispheres. The vestibular system keeps track of your overall sense of body position, movement and acceleration. Of course, this is usually all subconscious, but after a stroke, survivors have to retrain the brain to recognize this. Exercise is the best way to get it back.

CHAPTER 12

NUMBNESS AND LOSS OF SENSATIONS

C hanges in sensation are one of the first things that people notice when they are having a stroke, particularly numbness in the limbs on one side of the body or one side of the face. Often a survivor does not remember anything but waking up in the hospital unable to move their body after the stroke. By the time we meet them, they still may not feel parts of their face when they touch it as well as parts of their arm, hand, leg and foot on their affected side.

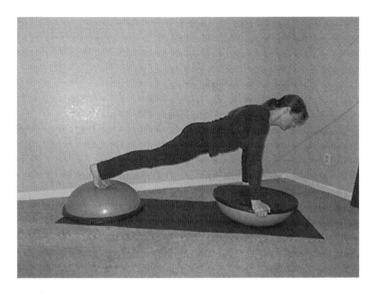

I had the incredible experience of being with a client when he was in the middle of an exercise and he stopped and said, "The sensation just came back in my hand." At this time, he was about two years post stroke, and he was able to do a plank while using two BOSU® balls. He had his hands holding onto one BOSU® ball as his feet were on the other BOSU® ball balancing in a plank. He stopped and said, "My feeling just came back in my hand." I asked him, "What do you mean?" He said, "I knew my hand was holding onto the BOSU® ball, but I never felt the sensation of touching it before now." We then walked to the front desk of the gym, and he got a water bottle out of the fridge and said, "I can feel the water is cold. I usually know I am holding the water bottle, but I had no idea the feeling of touching the bottle or the sensation of the hot or cold." This is known as cutaneous sensation. Cutaneous senses include touch and everything else we feel through our skin such as temperature, texture, pressure, vibration and pain. These receptors also sense whether the surface is hot or cold. This was a powerful moment.

CHAPTER 13

LEG BRACE, FOOT DROP AND TURN OUT

Almost every stroke survivor who has the foot drop is sent home wearing a leg brace on the lower portion of the leg on the affected side. These braces are called Ankle Foot Orthosis, known as AFOs. They are to keep the lower leg, ankle and foot stable enough for walking as well as controlling the foot drop and turn out, after a stroke.

The problem I have found personally with survivors is that it limits that part of the leg to recover. Repetitive and consistent movement and use to the area needing recovery won't take place if the brace is on forever. Depending on the strength of a client and their ability, I will ask them to remove it (if they are comfortable), so I can access the foot movement and their whole-body strength and weakness with it off. If it is possible and safe for the client, I will have them train under my watch of course, without their AFO on and have them continue to wear it when they know they need it for safety. Understanding that each survivor is different and are facing their own level of loss and challenges, one may always use an AFO while others may be able to stop using it. Most of my survivors have done away with the AFO and regained a proper foot step and walking gait.

As I mentioned before, I highly recommend finding a professional who has studied strokes and the biomechanics and movement of the human body. Working with foot drop is a perfect example why. The movement of the foot and lower leg in walking is not just based on the foot. It is based from a stable pelvic, which comes from a strong core, proper posture and the vastus muscles, especially the vastus medialis. See illustration as well as understand the importance of the sciatica nerve.

I give the client an option to remove it. I don't tell them they have to. I explain to them that it will limit the recovery of all that is needed for the proper use of that lower leg and foot usage to come back. Always be sure **safety** is the first concern. Not all survivors are ready to do this or are capable of doing this. Make your decision based on the strength of the rest of their body, coordination and walking and/or standing ability.

I am not a physical therapist, but I have found as I researched and in personal experience training with many stroke survivor clients, the brace does not help build any functional, structural strength needed to fix the problem.

When a survivor has a stronger core, which leads to stronger pelvic and stabilization this may be the best time to train without the AFO. Some research suggests that some strokes paralyze the vastus muscle group. Using the leg extension machine is one way to isolate the vastus muscle group. Note that this leg extension machine might be difficult for some survivors.

I start with a very light weight at 10-15 pounds. It can be extremely difficult. Take note of each individual client. Some may still be partially numb and very weak in their affected leg, especially in this particular movement. It may be easier for them to perform it well in full range of motion. Often when the focus is keeping the range of the movement by staying at the top 1/3. It may be extremely tough. Having the client try to keep the foot from turning out and to keep the toes towards them (dorsiflexion) may be more difficult. A couple of clients have told me that when I have had them position the foot dorsiflexed, it felt like I tripled the weight resistance compared to when the foot was in plantar flexion. Time this exercise so they can rest afterwards because it is quite fatiguing. Depending on the client, I have them work up to performing two to four sets of eight to ten reps. I base it on their energy level of that day.

Survivors need to watch their posture as they stand and sit. Remember not to slouch in poor posture with the recovery leg falling out to the side and foot turned out. This is teaching them to have awareness of where the foot is in space and what it is doing. They will have a harder challenge, if the rest of the day they continue to hold that foot and their posture in the position they are trying to fix when upright, standing and walking.

The body gets stronger in the movements and positioning it repeats most often. When there is a foot drop and leg turn out, it puts an imbalance up to the hip and to the spine. This is just as important to understand as knowing that having stable core and pelvis help keep the hips, knees, and feet in better alignment for best performance. Survivors need to be conscious (if they are able) of what the recovery leg and foot are doing as often as possible. In time, if they constantly remind themselves, they will begin to be aware. Ultimately, they will be able to move properly without thinking about it.

All the exercises combined can help bring walking gait to normal. Of course, doing them consistently and repeatedly is necessary.

As the fitness professional, it is best for us not to refer to the recovery leg as the "bad leg" as well as encouraging the survivor to be kind to the affected side. As mentioned in the communication chapter, we should encourage the survivor to be kind to the affected side.

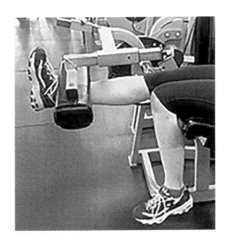

Dorsiflexion

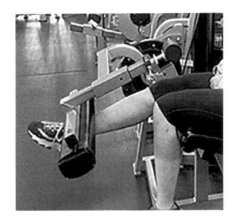

Plantar Flexion

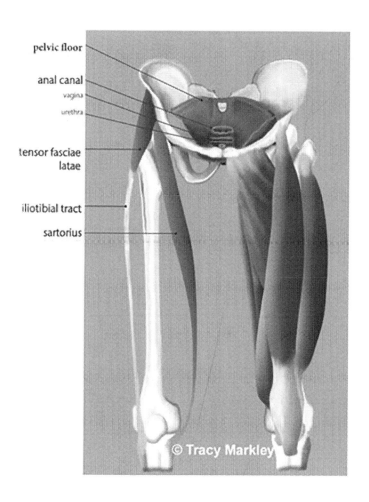

pelvic floor

anal canal

vagina

urethra

tensor fasciae latae

iliotibial tract

sartorius

© Tracy Markley

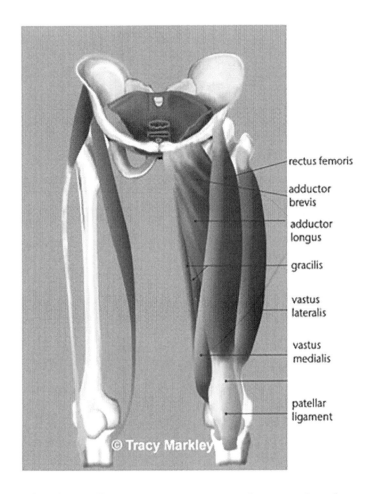

rectus femoris

adductor brevis

adductor longus

gracilis

vastus lateralis

vastus medialis

patellar ligament

© Tracy Markley

The above illustration is to give another visual to the muscles that need strengthened and possible new neuro pathways built for movement to come back.

Exercises. Sitting on ball with Bender® ball

Core/hip stabilization.

Standing on disc/BOSU® ball, stepping up and down.

Leg extension, 1/3 only at top.

Being aware of foot and hip placement, while standing sitting and walking.

Wear shoes with good ankle support.

No old shoes or loose, sloppy shoe tongues and laces.

A good resource about the AFOs

http://flintrehab.com/2017/afos-for-foot-drop-after-stroke/

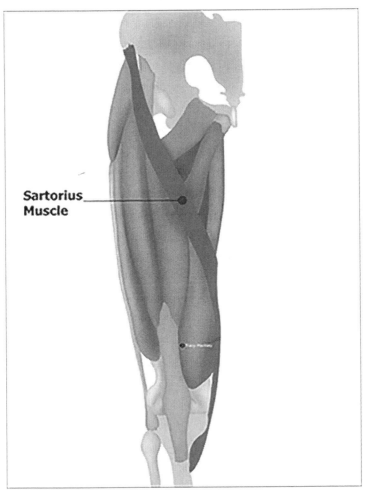

Sartorius Muscle

I share this illustration to teach that each muscle has its purpose for a movement and/or to help assist in a movement with other muscles. The more survivors, caregivers and professionals understand this, the greater chance to a stronger recovery.

The sartorius is the longest muscle in the body. The sartorius is attached to the front of the ilium, crosses over the medial side of the thigh and from the knee to the front of the tibia. Although it is an anterior muscle, it inserts into the tibia from behind the knee and it flexes the foreleg. It also flexes, abducts and laterally rotates the thigh at the hip. The more survivors, caregivers and professionals know about the muscles of the body and the movements they perform, the better chance of strengthening the body appropriately to help in further and stronger recovery.

CHAPTER 14

POSTURE IS
IMPORTANT

The client in my first book was an artist. He spent a great deal of his life with his shoulders rounded and his head forward. This is known as Kyphosis posture, and it contributed to the rotator cuff injury he had. He had many challenges when we began training together. He was six months post stroke and in a walker. He also had a rotator cuff injury that he had before he had his stroke.

We had some work to do to correct this, but it is impossible to rehab a shoulder properly if the thoracic spine and shoulder girdle are not staying in proper alignment. The stabilizing muscles of the body have to be strong enough to stabilize the rib cage, diaphragm and thoracic spine. This proper posture is necessary to keep the shoulder girdle in proper alignment, so the rotator cuff muscles can heal and rebuild correctly to keep the shoulder stable. This then leads to the head being able to stabilize in proper alignment. Poor posture causes the body to have mechanical deficiency and slow down motor control. It can cause physiological and neurological stress. Rounded shoulders and poor posture also affect the thoracolumbar fascia.

In addition, we were dealing with the effects of the stroke that left his arm feeling weak, heavy, numb and not taking commands from the brain for movements like it used to do.

We would work on the shoulder a bit, but there was not enough movement and stability to do this yet. He did go to the physical therapist for this in the beginning, but it was not working because he did not have the stability and strength in his core to hold his body upright in the correct posture to rebuild it. The body has a shoulder girdle and a shoulder joint. They are two different things. If the shoulder girdle is not held in its proper position for shoulder stabilization, the shoulder joint movement will be faulty. I wanted to build the body with proper mechanics for whole body performance and to avoid injuries now and in the future. Poor posture and body mechanics slow down motor control. We needed to speed up his motor control not slow it down.

After a year of working together, he had gained enough core strength and stability that when he went back to the therapist for the rotator cuff injury, it had begun to heal properly. I strongly believe it was because by that time, his core was strong enough that he was able to hold his shoulder girdle in proper alignment. This allowed the therapy exercises to ultimately work.

If someone does not have strong enough stabilizing muscles to hold the body upright, the shoulders are not going to be able to stay in proper alignment. It is biomechanics of the body. It is like piling a stack of boxes on top of one another. If the bottom box is half-full and unstable, everything that stacks on top begins to sink into the bottom box. They are unstable and out of balance, therefore they are unsafe and may fall.

When the head is balanced on the body correctly, you have better balance. If the core and rib cage are unstable, the shoulders cannot sit strongly in proper placement. Sitting on machines and working the upper back is not the cure for poor posture. It is important to strengthen the muscles at that angle as well, but there is more to it, as I just explained. It is crucial to understand muscle facilitation and recruitment patterns for the entire body. If posture is corrected, a client can do their exercises in the proper position and remain injury free. This also means when they exercise chest, biceps and triceps, they will be in their correct position. They can now do some functional exercises and can build up healthy recruitment patterns throughout the body without creating an injury or malfunction.

Approximately two years of posture changes shown as he is standing on the balance disc.

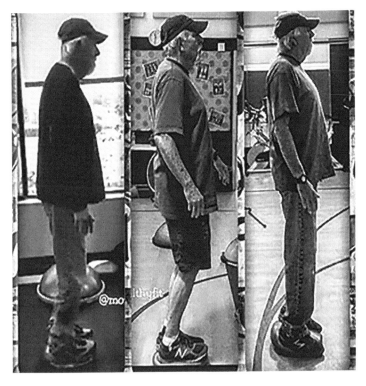

In the third picture you can see there is something on his hat. I sometimes use a small bean bag and place it on a client's head, to help him or her stand up tall. I use this often when helping clients walk. Not only are they focusing on keeping upright, so they do not drop the bean bag, it also gives them a sense of where their head is in space, spatial awareness. This is done when I know they are safe to do it. See my YouTube channel (Tracy

L. Markley Fitness) for a great example of the bean bag guiding a survivor to stand up tall when trying to walk. You will notice he had the awareness to where his head was in space by feeling the bean bag on his head and the natural instinct of not wanting it to fall off.

CHAPTER 15

SPASTICITY

Spasticity is high tone or activity in the muscles that makes them feel stiff and tight. Muscle spasticity **will tend to get worse the less the survivor moves**. The body must move to heal from a stroke. It is important to move as much as possible. Spasticity is one of the most common post-stroke conditions. If left untreated, spasticity can cause bone and joint deformities that are painful and debilitating. More than half of all stroke survivors do not seek treatment for spasticity

How Stroke Causes Spasticity

Muscles have a certain amount of tone or activity. The tone of muscles is controlled by signals from the brain. If the part of your brain that sends these control signals is damaged by a stroke, then the muscle may become too active. This is called spasticity.

About 30 percent of stroke survivors will experience some form of muscle spasticity. Some people experience spasticity immediately after their stroke, but it can start at any time.

Effects of Muscle Spasticity

Muscle spasticity can cause:

- Stiffness in the fingers, arms or legs.

- Muscle spasms.

- Overactive reflexes.

- Uncontrollable rhythmic contractions and relaxations in the muscles that lead to jerking. This is called clonus.

- Changes in posture. They may have spasticity in the psoas or another deep core muscle affecting one side and causing their spine to curve to one side.

- Pain.

Stroke survivors experiencing muscle spasticity may have:

- A clenched fist.

- A bent elbow and arm pressed against their chest.

- A stiff knee.

- A pointed foot.

- When attempting to move the stroke affected foot or hand, the upper body contracts and or swings forward to help.

Spasticity in leg muscles can make it difficult to walk. It can affect a survivor's balance and increase their risk of falling. Muscle spasticity can also increase tiredness or fatigue because it is harder to move. This also uses more energy and will cause the survivor to become more fatigued.

Common changes to arm and hand function may include:

- Weakness and paralysis
  The shoulder, elbow, wrist or hand may be weak, or they might not be able to move them. Hemiparesis is when you have weakness all the way down one side of your body. Hemiplegia is when one side of the body is paralyzed.

- Sensation
  Survivors might lose feeling in their arm or hand, and experience numbness or "pins and needles." Alternatively, they might have hypersensitivity or increased feeling, which can make even light touch painful.

- Coordination
  If the affected arm doesn't move in the way they want it to, they may have apraxia (also known as dyspraxia). This is when they have difficulty planning or coordinating movements.

- Swelling
  Fluid might build up in their hand or arm

when it doesn't move as well as it used to. This is called edema.

- Muscle tone
  High muscle tone, called hypertonia or spasticity, makes a muscle stiff or tight. Low muscle tone, or hypotonia, makes a muscle floppy or loose.

- Subluxation
  The shoulder joint can become partially or incompletely dislocated. This happens when weakness or low muscle tone causes the top of the arm to drop out of its socket.

- Contracture
  Muscle shortening due to weakness or high tone can make joints less flexible, or even become fixed in one position.

References:

The Spasticity Alliance
http://www.spasticityalliance.org

"The Stroke of An Artist, The Journey of a Fitness Trainer and a Stroke Survivor," by Tracy L. Markley

CHAPTER 16

PILATES

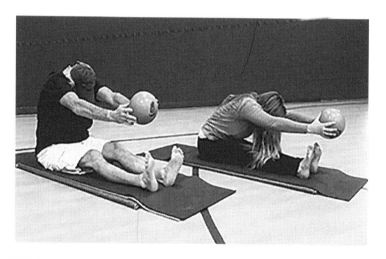

Pilates is another great resource in stroke recovery. Pilates focuses on stabilizing and strengthening the center of the body to transfer power to the limbs and arms and decreases stress on ligaments and joints. It improves mental strength. Pilates flows with fluidity and grace. Pilates trains whole-body integration that reflects healthy fascia throughout the body.

In Pilates, one should be focused on every movement, as they flow through each exercise. I began teaching every client to understand this mindset needed in stroke recovery, as they perform every exercise. It is difficult for many people to focus and be present when they exercise, but it is especially hard after one has a stroke.

I recommend a client use Pilates based on the Joseph Pilates method and to seek out a professional who has knowledge and/or a certification in the Joseph Pilates method.

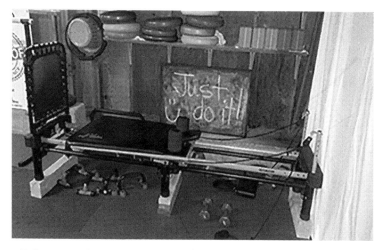

Pilates Reformer – this is a home version of a Reformer.

CHAPTER 17

PAIN

Some survivors may experience pain throughout their body. Some may have one painful area always. I find this to be more common in either a hip or a shoulder and sometimes both. Post-stroke pain can occur immediately, weeks or sometimes even months after a stroke. Research shows that more than half of stroke survivors have some form of post-stroke pain. In some cases, the pain is constant (chronic), and in others, it comes and goes. This is because the messages between the brain and nerves are confused, and the nerves are triggering pain.

Making new pathways of communication is part of the brain healing. Stimulating the brain and spinal column (the central nervous system), as the survivor performs their exercises to release the spasticity, can aid in the healing and recovery. If the brain sends a message to the multifidus muscle and the balancing system (as I like to call it) first before sending messages to the limbs, it makes sense to heal and strengthen the muscles involved in the balancing system. If this area is weak and out of sorts, it can be a road block to clear communication from the brain to the muscles. Remember consistency, receptiveness and patience is involved in recovery.

There is also central post-stroke pain (CPSP)— an effect of stroke where the person has painful burning, throbbing or shooting feelings, although there is nothing present that would normally cause pain. Doctors may call this thalamic pain syndrome because it can be caused by damage to the part of the brain called the thalamus. While there is no cure for central post-stroke pain, some medicines can help manage it.

We may not know the exact cause of the pain, but we try to help them the best we can, by helping them recover as much of their body movement, posture and balance as we can. This often helps the pain go away.

I find there are many avenues of exercise that different therapists have patients perform for their hand and arm therapy. I have clients stand on a balance disc or BOSU® ball, if possible and safe for them, to perform these exercises. In therapy often, I give the patient something to squeeze. I like to have the survivor work on extension and opening motions of the hand, while on the unstable surfaces of the disc and BOSU® ball. In time, if done consistently, that clenching, tight hand begins to release.

There are many options survivors try. There are options for Botox or phenol injections and some may have possible surgery options and intrathecal baclofen pump therapy. Some say these options work, others say they don't. I say as with many things, if it works, do it. If it does not work, try something else. Each survivor is unique to their own recovery. Persistence and patience are key.

Most likely, trying an exercise a couple times a week will not bring the healing one hopes for. Exercises need to be done almost daily and often. The body was made to move and it needs to try to do a movement repeatedly for the brain to make a new pathway. The brain is trying. Remember the brain needs to be hydrated, nourished and stimulated to aid in its healing.

Resources and more information
https://www.saebo.com/pain-stroke-symptoms-watch The Spasticity Alliance http://www.spasticityalliance.org

Tracy L. Markley Fitness and Author
YouTube Channel
https://youtu.be/fF6blukxpAA

CHAPTER 18

VISION AND PERIPHERAL VISION LOSS

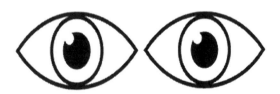

It is common for many stroke patients to have a loss of peripheral vision on one side. I conducted an experiment with a client who was having great physical gains. I thought if all these gains and progress in his condition were happening, maybe it could work as well on his peripheral vision loss. I spoke to a mentor of mine, and he supposed that no one had tried it, so it wasn't known if it could help or not. He encouraged me to go for it and see what happened.

I began by holding different objects and having him track them with his eyes, as I moved the objects. Sometimes I would have him follow with his eyes without moving his head and other times moving his head. At our next visit, I grabbed items around the gym in different colors. I found things blue, red, green, purple, orange and yellow. I then discovered he could not see colors correctly. It took at least 15 seconds to a minute before he would say a color, and a couple colors were not registering in his brain at all. I then thought, "Let's have him stand on the balance disc!" To our great surprise, his brain registered some of the colors almost instantly. Standing on an unstable surface, such as the balance disc, stimulates the central nervous system.

This helped me understand that the stimulation of the brain and the nervous system could do such a thing. This was an experience that clearly confirmed that both of these unstable surfaces, the balance disc and the BOSU® ball, stimulate the nervous system at a level I was not aware of. This helped me understand that because of the client's fragile neurological state, I was able to actually see, and not just be aware, that the nervous system was being stimulated. The next day, I brought in different colored construction paper, and we began working on seeing colors as he stood on the balance disc for 10 minutes each session. It was incredible to witness such dynamics.

At times, it was frustrating for him because he would see a color but would say a different color. Once I told him the correct color, he would explain how he knew it, but the brain was not processing the right color he wanted to say. Since he had been an artist his whole life, his brain would try to identify the exact shade of blue as we see in paint and crayons. It was definitely a lot of work for his brain.

At this time, he was still working on getting quicker movements and reaction time with his arms and hands. This is when I suggested that he get the

Simon® game and use it at home when he was on the disc. Simon® is an electronic memory game that came out in the 1980s and is still in stores. It has four big buttons to press, and they are all different colors. The game makes a different noise with each flashing color, and you have to follow the pattern with memory. The idea was for him to stand on the balance disc and have the Simon® game to the side that was affected by the stroke. This would help stimulate his brain, help regain faster reaction time and help his memory.

Visual tracking also helps with spatial awareness and balance, especially if they are able to stand on an unstable surface while doing it. Visual tracking is following an object with the eyes. It can be done with just the eyes and leaving the head still or turning the head to follow the object. The client can do this alone or with assistance.

You may find that the survivors with spasticity on their affected side will be unable to do this on their own. They will need a trainer or a caregiver to help them.

CHAPTER 19

FULL BODY WORKOUTS

It is important to work the full body if possible. As we continue to understand the human body and movement, we know that a muscle does not work alone to make a movement. Certain muscles help stabilize the body as other muscles are being activated to perform a specific movement. The brain needs to be retrained to multitask the nervous systems, the muscular system and fascial system throughout the whole body, because that is how the body naturally works. We need to do the isolated work. For example, working on the hand opening up when fighting their spasticity in their hand, but doing this as they stand on the balance disc or BOSU® ball, if possible, will help bring it back faster.

When you think how the right lat muscles work in movement with the left gluteal muscles, it also makes sense as to why working the full body, not just the affected side, will bring greater recovery results for the survivor.

I conducted a survey that indicated many professionals have their clients work only their stroke-affected side and not the entire body. These clients usually have more limited recovery.

CHAPTER 20

BALANCE DISC - BOSU® BALL - SWISS BALL – BALANCE PAD

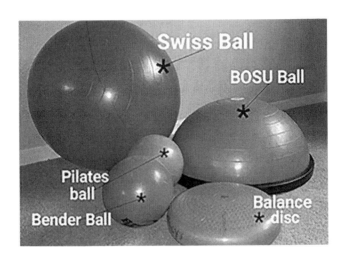

Swiss Ball

The Swiss ball was developed in 1963 by Aquilino Cosani, an Italian plastics manufacturer. A British physiotherapist used it in physical therapy in Switzerland. In the 1980s, physical therapists brought the Swiss ball to America, and soon it came into the fitness industry.

As years have passed, the Swiss ball has been labeled as an exercise ball, a yoga ball, a therapy ball and many other names. It is used for various exercises. I use it frequently in my workouts, and with clients.

It is a ball that is big enough to sit on, as shown in the pictures.

Important points when using this ball:

- Have the ball at a height where your hips DO NOT drop below the knees.

- Be sure the ball is firm. You will not get proper spine support if the ball is mushy when you sit on it or when you use it for exercises.

- Sit with your knees over the ankles, (shins straight up and down). You don't want to sink into the knee joints.

- Always begin with caution. When first using the ball keep yourself near something to hold onto for safety.

Bender® Ball

The Bender® ball is a 9-inch inflatable plastic exercise ball. Other 9-inch balls are available, and are often referred to as Pilates balls or small exercise balls. They usually all work. They come in a variety of rubber thicknesses. I have used the Bender® ball for years, and I know exactly what I am getting when I place an order for myself or a client.

Balance Disc & BOSU® Ball

The BOSU® ball is called a BOSU® Balance Trainer. Both the BOSU® ball and the balance disc are considered unstable surfaces. I use the balance disc and BOSU® ball with most clients. Balance discs are round, air-filled discs that are strong enough to sit, stand and exercise on. They are added to workouts to improve balance and increase core strength. The discs and the BOSU® ball are considered unstable environments to exercise on. They both challenge your balance, and they both stimulate the central nervous system, which is the brain and spinal column. I use the 13-inch balance discs with my clients.

The balance disc is referred to as an unstable-stable environment, whereas the BOSU® ball is referred to as a stable-unstable environment. It was scientifically invented to absorb the body's weight into its dome, allowing the bracing system in the body to relax. Therefore, the nerves are stimulated deeper into the nerve roots. Both these tools are fantastic to use at any age for many great advantages. I feel they are essential to use with my clients in order to gain the best functioning body. I share some basic balance and neurological exercises in this book. There are many other exercises that all the tools listed in this chapter can be used for.

Balance Disc

The balance disc is an air-filled stability wobble cushion. They usually come in different sizes. I usually use a 13-inch balance disc. I have used the balance discs with clients for almost 20 years to help strengthen the spine, core, posture, joints and ligaments. Standing on the balance disc and BOSU® balls also stimulates the central nervous system. Clients use them to strengthen their balancing. We used them to warm up the spine with various gentle exercises, while standing or kneeling on them. We would do some free weights, while standing or kneeling as well. I explained to clients that we were activating and strengthening the small deep muscles around the spine and working on the core and balance. We were stimulating the nervous system. As I worked with stroke survivors and clients with neurological challenges, I never experienced just how much was actually taking place neurologically, until the last few years when I began working with more clients with strong neurological issues. When clients made neurological changes, they were very visible.

The disc is known as an unstable, unstable surface and the BOSU® ball is known as a stable, unstable surface. The BOSU® ball was invented to absorb the body's weight into its dome, allowing the bracing system in the body to relax. Therefore, the nerves get stimulated deeper into the nerve roots. This is why my clients with neuropathy, plantar fasciitis, fascia issues and various neurological issues had shown significant, unexpected improvements when they used the BOSU® ball. Just standing on the BOSU® ball increases muscle strength. It is due to adaptation in the neurological system and the resistance through the lower body from standing on the BOSU® ball. It's not only considered a balance tool but a resistance tool. It is a 3-D pressurized, elastic resistance tool that you compress with the feet as you stand on it and do specific exercises properly.

Balance Pads

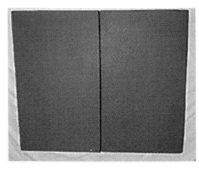 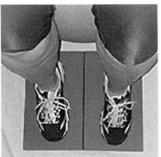

Balance pads are a mild unstable surface. They can be used for the same exercises as the disc and BOSU® ball. The pad would be used for those who cannot stand on the disc or BOSU® ball yet. I also use it to place on a chair to sit on as it helps make the chair height higher.

In the beginning of training some stroke survivors, they may not be able to be on the BOSU® ball because of its height and width. We need the client to be in control and stay safe while they step on and off of it. If they are challenged with the loss of spatial awareness and possible peripheral loss or blur on one side, they will have a harder time controlling their feet in placement. Standing and stepping off and on the BOSU® ball is excellent for survivors once they are safe to do it. I am not a physical therapist, nor do I have harnesses at my studio as they do in therapy facilities for safety. I have to rely on the client being able to step on and off safely and to hold on to the bar and maintain stability on their own, to avoid falls and injuries.

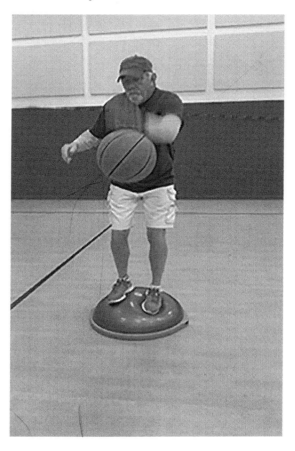

In this photo, the 67-year-old stroke survivor is two and one-half years post stroke. He is squatting up and down slowly on the BOSU® ball, as he is bouncing a basketball. This was possible after a year of just standing and balancing on the balance discs and BOSU® ball and stepping on and off the BOSU® ball. His persistence and consistency were incredible for his progress. Clients must be willing to be consistent and persistent to achieve such great gains. In the first-year of training with me, bouncing a ball was extremely frustrating for him. The coordination and hand control on the right side was not ready for such a task. As his spatial awareness, proprioception and different cognitive skills became stronger, he was able to coordinate all the skills needed to combine the BOSU® ball and bouncing the basketball. In this picture, his nervous system is being stimulated and fired up as there is resistance force going up his legs. He is balancing and coordinating where to bounce the ball and how high so he can still control his hands. There are many amazing internal things going on. This is one of his most incredible and my favorite combination of skills in an activity he achieved. This includes spatial awareness cognitive skills to coordinate the reach to the ball, the controlling of the arm and hand to how much speed and power was needed to get the ball to bounce to the height he wanted, as well as controlling it in his space so it did not hit the BOSU® ball instead of the floor. He was also able to do this as he was in movements of repeated squats. This looks like it was easy for this stroke survivor, but it was not. He could do it well, but it took one hundred percent focus and concentration. He did it; then he stepped off and said, "Wow, that is hard." We worked together over two years before he was ready to work on this.

This also meant many movements and cognitive skills needed for everyday life had also developed. This achievement, as in all of them, was a foundation for the next functional gain his body was going to attain to help him in everyday activities and movements.

CHAPTER 21

EXERCISES

Here are some important exercises I have found essential to regaining balance, strength and stability for safe movement. Depending on the client, I may have them start by sitting on a Swiss ball, standing on the balance disc, or I may have them start by standing on the BOSU® ball. In all cases, especially in the beginning, I have the client hold on to a ballet barre or the squat rack bar, even though I am in the fitness studio. If you are trying these at home, be sure to have a safe item to hold onto.

In each standing exercise:

- Engage the core. Imagine you are zipping up a zipper to put on a snug girdle.

- Be aware of your body's location in space from head to toe.

- Be aware of feet placement. Feel them evenly anchored wherever you are standing. Try to keep feet evenly placed, don't let them roll out to the sides.

- Stand up tall, stack the shoulders over the hips, and imagine you are lengthening your spine to the sky.

- Imagine your body weight is lifting up, as the feet maintain the sense of being anchored in the ground.

- For safety, if needed, hold onto a bar or secure object, which allows you to maintain a good posture.

- Hold on enough to be safe, but don't become so stiff that you don't feel the balancing challenge of the disc or BOSU® ball.

- If you are sitting on the stability (Swiss) ball, anchored as described above, keep the knees over the ankles, and sit up tall with your shoulders over your hips.

- Follow the instructions and tips listed with each of the following exercises.

Exercise 1

Sitting on a Stability (Swiss) Ball

- Be sure the ball is firm.

- Be sure the ball is the right height for you. (Your hips should be level with your knees. Do not sit on a mushy ball or on a ball where your hips are below your knees.)

- Sit on the ball so that your legs are as close to the ball as they can be without touching it.

- Keep your knees directly over your ankles. This means your shin bone will be in a straight line from the ankle to the knee. Think of table legs coming directly out of the table joint, which allows the table leg to be positioned straight up and down.

- Don't let your knees fall in or fall out, and don't squeeze your legs together.

- Anchor your feet into the floor.

- Engage your pelvic floor (if possible), without engaging the glutes (squeezing your butt muscles).

- Engage your core like you are putting on a snug girdle.

- Stack your shoulders over the hips.

In the beginning, a survivor may feel that there are too many things to remember. That is okay, it is normal. Keep focusing from head to toe. This will help the body and brain regain better communication consciously, which will help rebuild the communication subconsciously, as you strengthen the muscles in your spine and core.

A survivor's stroke affected leg may fall out to the side and they may not be able to hold a ball between their legs without assistance from their own hand or a professional. I like to have the survivor sit near a wall in a chair. I then place a ball between the wall and the affected leg. Then they can use another ball between the knees to do the exercise the best they can.

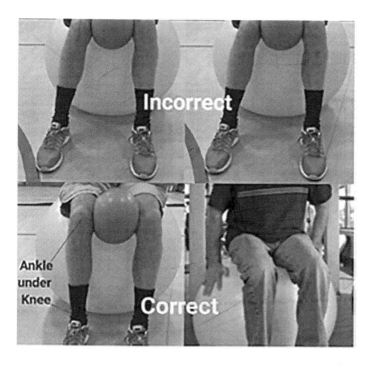

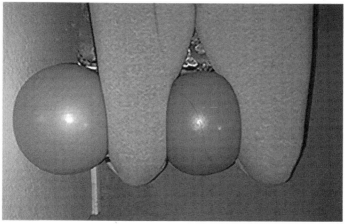

This picture is a bird's eye view of using both balls near a wall.

Exercise 2

Sitting on a Stability (Swiss) Ball - Adductor/Abductor Exercise

Use a Bender® ball or a small soft Pilates ball, and gently squeeze between the knees/inner thighs. This can be done with your feet flat on the floor and on tip toes.

- Set up your position on the ball, (as in Exercise 1).

- Place the ball between your knees or inner thighs, wherever it feels comfortable for you.

- Check your position and posture again and visualize yourself putting on that girdle, (as in Exercise 1).

- Gently but firmly squeeze the ball between your knees (inner thighs), with control, then release, with control. Repeat this movement for 10 to 20 reps. Be sure to use the same speed throughout the exercise. (Try NOT to squeeze the ball, and then quickly snap the release.) Work yourself up to three sets of 20 reps. This number changes and varies per person. When I am working with a client, we communicate and determine the number that works for them, together based on the strength and ability of the client.

- Do NOT engage the glutes (squeeze the buttocks) while performing this exercise. For most people, this takes focus.

- As with any exercises, if your back, hip or knee joints hurt while doing this exercise, first recheck your form and if that does not fix it, <u>STOP</u> the exercise!

- It is never a good idea to hurt one area of the body in order to strengthen another. Proper exercise that works for the whole body, while avoiding injuries, is essential.

Exercise 3

~~~~~~

Standing on the Balance Disc

It is important to have a balance disc that is not too flimsy. I have found that the CanDo® brand 35cm/13 inch is a good one to use.

- Engage the core. Imagine you are zipping up a zipper to put on a snug girdle before even stepping onto the balance disc. Re-engage once you are standing on the balance disc.

- Be aware of the body's location in space from head to toe.

- Be aware of feet placement. Feel them evenly anchored where you are standing. Try to keep your feet evenly placed, don't let them roll out to the sides.

- Stand up tall, stack your shoulders up over your hips and imagine you are reaching the top of your head to the sky.

- Imagine your body weight is lifting up as your feet maintain the sense of being anchored to the ground.

- Hold onto a bar or secure object so you can maintain a good posture, but don't hold the body so stiff that you don't feel the balancing challenge of the disc.

- Depending on each survivor's balance strength or challenges, they have to begin at their own level.

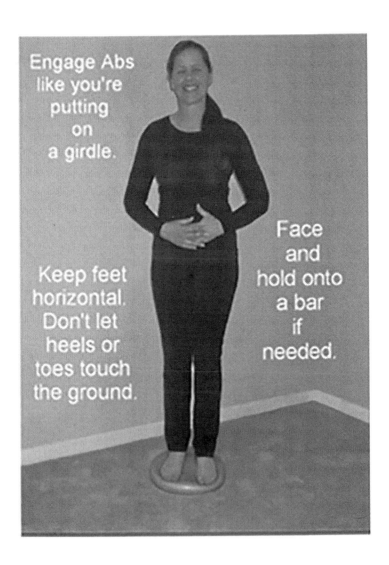

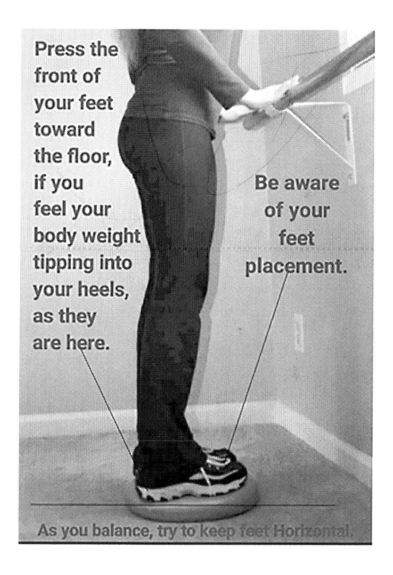

Press the front of your feet toward the floor, if you feel your body weight tipping into your heels, as they are here.

Be aware of your feet placement.

As you balance, try to keep feet Horizontal.

153

Exercise 4

^^^

Standing on the BOSU® Ball

It is important that you have the BOSU® ball inflated to its proper firmness. Usually, if you turn the BOSU® ball over so that the platform is facing up and measure the distance from the floor to the top of the platform, it should be about 9 to 10 inches off the ground. I have noticed that BOSU® balls can vary a bit in size. A flatter ball DOES NOT MEAN IT'S A BETTER CHALLENGE. That is not how it works, it is not the science behind this piece of equipment.

- Engage the core. Imagine you are zipping up a zipper to put on a snug girdle before even stepping up from the floor. Re-engage once, standing on the BOSU® ball.

- Be aware of your body's location in space from head to toe.

- Be aware of feet placement. Feel them evenly anchored to where you are standing.

Try to keep your feet evenly placed, and don't let them roll out to the sides.

- Stand up tall, stack your shoulders up over your hips and imagine you are reaching the top of your head to the sky.

- Imagine that your body weight is lifting up, as your feet maintain the sense of being anchored.

- Hold onto a bar or secure object so that you can maintain good posture, but don't hold the body so stiff that you don't feel the balancing challenge of the BOSU® ball.

- Depending on your individual balance strength or challenges, you have to begin at your own level.

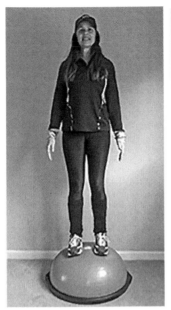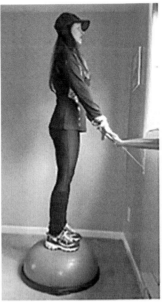

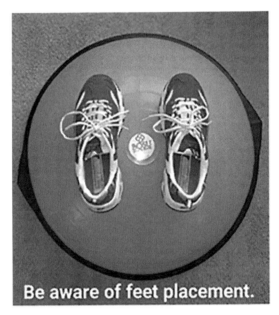

Be aware of feet placement.

Exercise 5

Stepping on and off the BOSU® Ball

- Engage as explained in Exercise 1 or for the balance disc before even stepping onto the dome of the BOSU® ball.

- Spend a few minutes standing and balancing.

- When you are ready to step up and down, remind yourself to stay focused, and mindful of each individual foot's placement, as you step up and step down.

- Come to a complete balance, once both feet are on the dome. Stand up tall, stacking your shoulders over your hips.

- When you feel balanced, stay focused, and then step back to the floor.

- Once you come to a complete balance on the floor, stand up tall, stacking your shoulders over your hips. Then step back onto the dome.

- If possible, begin by stepping up with the right foot and stepping down with the right foot. Do these five times; then switch to stepping up with the left foot and stepping down with the left foot.

- Work yourself up to 10 on each side.

- If you personally have a foot drag, a drop challenge or another physical challenge or weakness making this difficult to do, *KEEP PRACTICING.* It will get easier with time. *The more you are receptive to a movement, the better chance the brain has of making the new pathway needed for such a movement.*

- When stepping off to the floor, focus on clearing the dome. The goal is not to let your foot drag down the dome or hit the plastic platform. If you have extra physical challenges, this movement will come with time. *KEEP PRACTICING.*

- When finished with stepping up and down, go back to just standing and balancing. You will find you can balance better now. If the first few times you don't experience this, it will come with time. *KEEP PRACTICING.*

This is a very important exercise to help you regain balance and rebuild a safe and strong walking gait. It helps to rebuild an awareness of the location of your feet in space during your movement.

We take small steps stepping backwards many times each day:

-When we open a door towards us.

-When we approach a chair to sit down.

-Doing laundry.

-Stepping down a ladder or step.

-Backing away from the bathroom or kitchen sink.

-Using your feet to push yourself in a chair away from a table before you stand and more.

If you are having a hard time with the exercise of walking backwards, begin with Exercise 5 first, and/or include it in your workout program before you work on walking backward.

*Remember, the brain sends a message to the deep core muscles to stabilize the body before movement. Exercise 5 will help rebuild the body's natural system of flow for stepping and walking backward.

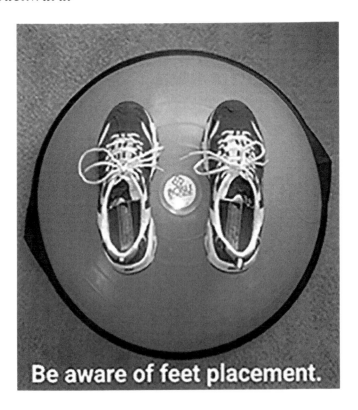

Be aware of feet placement.

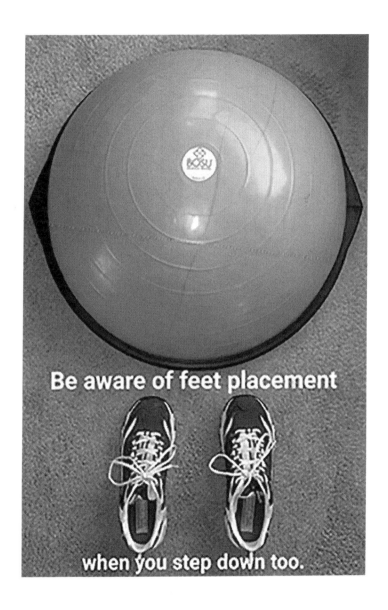

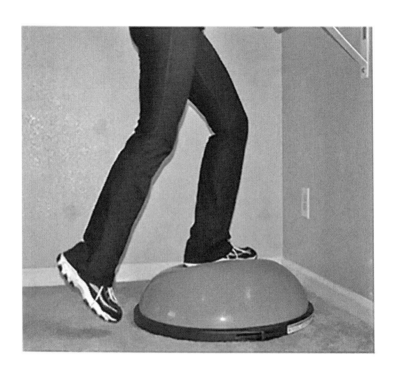

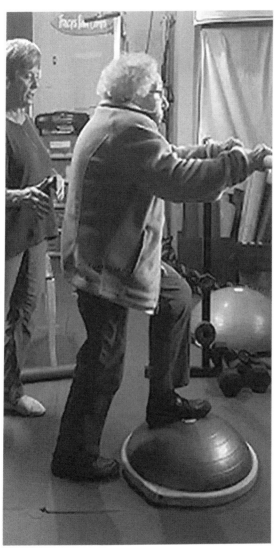

*If they are unable to step on the standard BOSU®
ball, have them use a child size BOSU® ball, if they
are able. The client in this photo was only 4 feet 11.*

Exercise 6

∿∿∿∿∿∿∿∿∿∿∿∿∿∿∿∿∿∿∿∿∿∿∿∿∿∿∿∿∿∿

Walking Across Thee or More BOSU® Balls

This is more advanced.

Only do this exercise when you are stable enough to do it!

- Begin with placing the BOSU® balls in a straight line next to a barre. Use a ballet barre or a squat rack bar at the gym that holds the rack securely in place, or use something secure.

- Hold on safely with one hand, facing the end of the row of domes.

- Engage your core, and be aware of your body from head to toe as explained in previous exercises.

- When you are ready, step up on the first dome.

- Find your balance and stand up tall, staying engaged.

- When ready, safely step from the first dome onto the second dome.

- When you are balanced and feel in control, safely step onto the third dome.

- Find your balance again, and when feeling safe and in control, step off the dome onto the floor.

- Turn around and repeat, going in the other direction. (You are now holding on with the other hand.)

- Depending on each individual, if you are more challenged on one side and are having a hard time holding on with a particular hand, do not walk on domes in that direction until you feel safe and/or have a therapist or qualified professional with you.

- Try stepping from one dome to the next, leading with the right foot for some steps. Then do the same, leading with the left foot.

- Start focused, try to control the step of each foot, and place it exactly where you want it to be.

- Do not randomly land your foot anywhere. Work on controlling your step.

- *Advanced.* **If** and **only when** you are ready, instead of stepping on to the floor to turn around, turn around on the last dome very slowly, with very small steps and with control.

- *Advanced.* **If** and **only when** you are ready, walk across the domes without holding onto a barre/bar. Remember, it is not necessary to do this without holding onto something in order to achieve results.

Incorporating BOSU® Balls

Standing on a BOSU® ball is extremely good for balance, stability, walking, awareness of feet placement, quick reaction time, the neurological system, strengthening the core, pelvic and leg muscles, focus and more. In time, a client may begin to step from one ball to the other and possibly do a squat and then step to the next. As seen in the exercise section of this book, have client hold onto a bar of some sort for safety, until they are ready not to use a bar. They may always have to use the bar, and that is okay. In time they may begin to turn around on the last ball and go back across them instead of stepping on the floor to turn around. This may take months of practice and may never be perfected, but the outcome in strength, coordination, balance and brain exercise is still taking place.

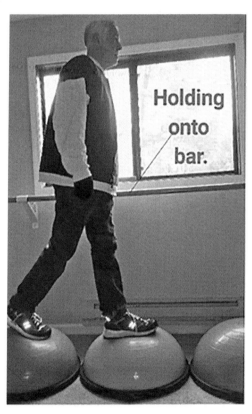

Holding onto bar.

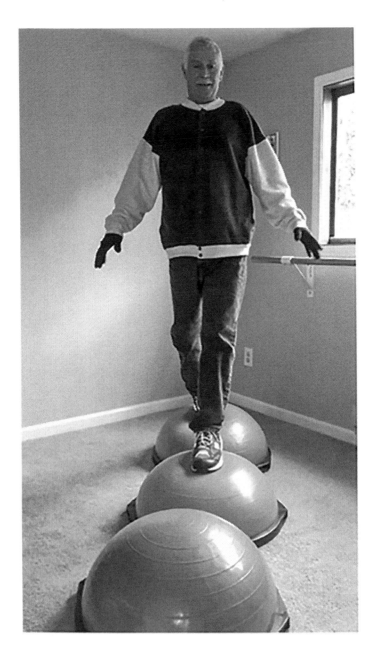

Exercise 7

Walking Backward

Only practice walking backward, if client can safely do so.

Client can walk alongside a bar, or something to hold onto if needed.

If client does not have control of placing each foot exactly where they want it when they step, <u>walking backward will not be safe for them to do.</u> <u>Safety first.</u>

After doing the previous exercises for some time, the ability to walk backward will feel safe again.

Once a client is ready to walk backward, find a safe area. I find it is best to have a mirror in front of a client, if possible, to watch themselves, but this is not always an available option.

If client is using a walker, DO THIS ONLY in a safe space with a professional guiding them.

The picture below is my 105-year-old client walking toward the mirror forward, then walking backward as she still faced the mirror. Her posture is nice and strong from our work together. She was amazing.

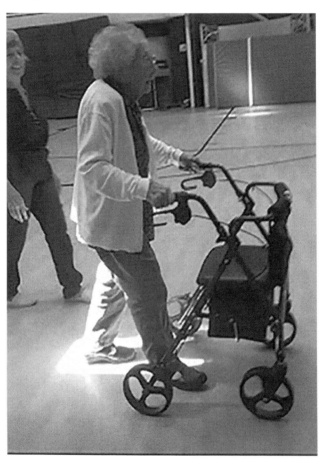

Exercise 8

Squats Holding on to a Bar

This exercise can be done standing on the floor or standing on the BOSU® ball.

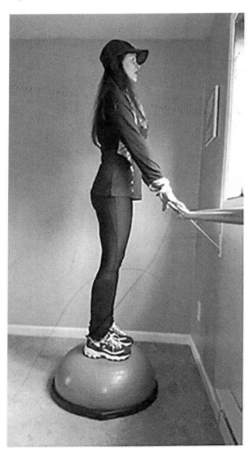

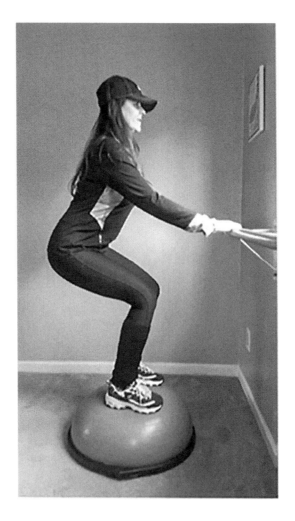

- Begin by doing this exercise with your feet on the floor first to be sure you can hold the proper alignment safely before you begin performing this on the dome of the BOSU®

ball. You can also do this standing on a balance pad as you are becoming stronger to squat with the BOSU® ball.

- While facing the bar, evenly hold on to the bar with your hands, so that your body is centered between your hands.

- Engage your core, and focus. Hold the body in good form from head to toe, including the shoulders.

- Sit back as if you are going to sit in a chair, then raise yourself back up.

- Try to use your legs and glutes to do the movement. Don't allow the arms to do all the work.

- Do not drop the hips below the knees.

- If this bothers your knees, check your form. If it still bothers your knees do not do the exercise.

- If you are doing this standing on the floor, pull yourself up to a good posture between each squat.

- If you are doing this on the dome, pull yourself up to good posture, and balance yourself straight up and down in good form between each squat.

- Maintain control and focus throughout each movement.

- In each squat, make sure both feet are parallel, so that your hips and pelvis are moving evenly through both sides throughout each rep.

- If you are using the BOSU® ball, do about 8-10 squats, then spend a couple of minutes balancing on the dome. When you are stronger, work up to three sets of 10 squats, balancing in between.

- Work your way up to the squatting. Depending on each individual, you may not feel safe to do the squats in the first few weeks.

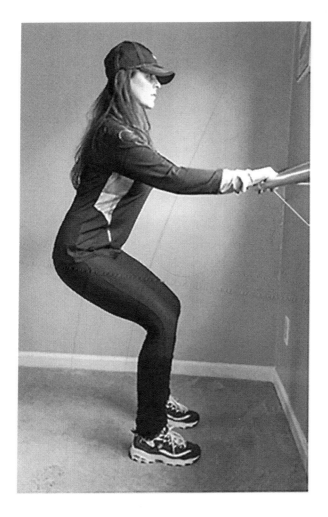

Practice walking forward every day. Practice all of these exercises daily if you can. Listen to your body and its guidance.

These are the basic exercises used with all the clients whose stories I've shared throughout this book. If you jumped straight to the exercise chapter of this book and skipped the stories of the client's journeys, I encourage you strongly to go back and read each story.

The body needs to heal. Each person's body heals at its own pace. Try to be patient and respect your own body. Be kind to yourself.

When you feel ready to add some free weights, you can sit on the Swiss ball, stand on the disc, stand on the BOSU® ball or even kneel on the BOSU® ball and do bicep curls, shoulder raises or other upper body exercises in proper form. I don't suggest doing overhead exercises when you are using these unstable surfaces, it can put pressure on your spine.

Stay safe.

If needed while standing on disc or BOSU® ball, hold on with one hand while doing a bicep curl in the other hand. This technique can be used with any specific exercise that the client can do safely and effectively one side at a time.

Often in the beginning, one side will be harder to hold on with. Monitor each client individually to what they can and cannot do. This can be done sitting on a ball or in a chair if needed, as well. Be sure the whole body is in the best posture it can be in from head to toes.

The more a survivor can do exercises as they are on the Swiss ball, BOSU® ball, balance disc or balance pad, the whole body will be working and challenged for movement, balance and functional training. This is what is needed for everyday life.

Survivors can work on one side at a time to help with spasticity in the arms, hands and fingers. Have them focus on the hand that is not affected by the stroke. Focus, concentrate with eyes open and closed, visualize in the mind and feel what that hand is doing, so when they go to train on the stroke affected side, they can use the visualization and focus that is used on the non-affected side. Do this sitting, until able to do on an uneven surface as on the disc and BOSU® ball.

Exercise 9

~~~~~~

Battling Ropes

Battling ropes, also called battle ropes, are a great tool for stroke survivors and clients with balance and neurological challenges. They work well for neuro-rehabilitation for stroke, brain injuries and cardiac rehab clients and excellent for age related disease. Battle ropes have low risk of injury and are non-impact weight resistance. There is a two-vector force direction created, while using the battle ropes. This means one direction of force is pulling away from the client, while a downward force from the pull of gravity from the weight of the ropes. This causes multiple contractions of different muscle groups at the same time. At the same time, they challenge the dynamic balance and stabilization while using them. They are being used more and more for rehabilitation and corrective exercises. They help clients with asymmetrical stabilization issues. Depending on the recovery stage in a client, one may only use one rope at a time or two ropes at a time. There are different wave patterns to use with the ropes that create velocity, and they challenge the core muscles in different patterns.

Ropes can be used by clients in wheelchairs and walkers. They can be seated in their wheelchairs or on a chair that is an appropriate height for their height and hip level. They can be used sitting on a ball, standing on the floor and standing and sitting on the BOSU® ball, squatting, lunging, kneeling and more. I took a Battling Rope Coach Certification course with NESTA to better my knowledge, while using the ropes with clients. There is much more to battling ropes then I am mentioning in this book.

There are hundreds of exercises that can be done with them. They come in different lengths, diameters and weight of the ropes. A few basic tips. Understand the purpose of the different hand grips. Keep the client in proper posture. Have the shoulder girdles set in proper alignment.

A survivor may be able to use both ropes at once or a single rope. It will depend on the individual challenges they are working through. The way the hands grip the battle ropes make a difference. If a client has an arm that won't work well with the ropes yet, use a single rope with the double hand grip. If possible, perform the exercises in one position; then rotate the hands, so the other hand is on top, and perform the exercises again. The stronger arm of course will be in control, but the other arm will follow in movement and participate in the exercise as well, but with guidance with the other hand. I suggest having the client perform making waves with the battle ropes and the tsunamis. These can be done standing or kneeling on the ground, sitting in a chair, wheelchair, roller walker, Swiss ball, standing and sitting on the BOSU® ball.

Different Hand Grips May Be Used While Using Battle Ropes.

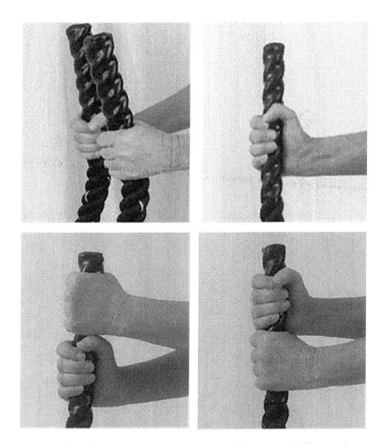

In this hand grip, as the client performs Waves or the Tsunamis exercises with the battle ropes, the push muscles are being worked

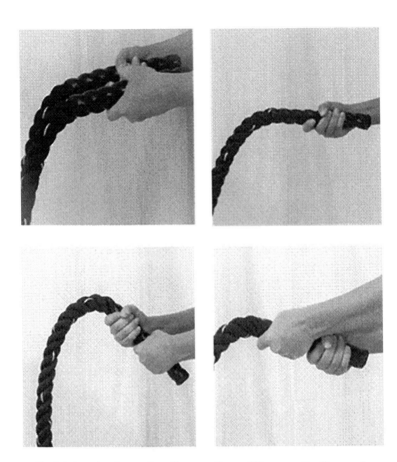

In this hand grip, as the client performs Waves or the Tsunamis exercises with the battle ropes, the pull muscles are being worked

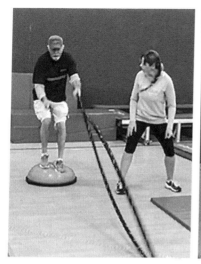
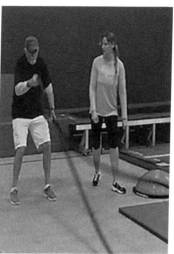

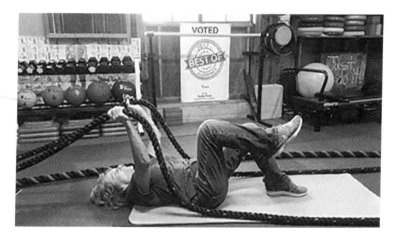

Combining battle ropes with some Pilates ab exercises is also a great source, if the survivor's arms/shoulders can do it. In this exercise, the ropes are wrapped securely around a pole. This client is keeping shoulders in place, abs engaged as she slowly lifts one leg and lowers it back down with control. She moves at the same speed for both directions. Combining with the ropes as she is, she is strengthening the core, arms and shoulder stabilization. These are 30-pound 30-foot ropes. They come in different lengths, diameters and weights.

The ropes are also usually fun for the clients. There are many exercises that can be done with them. It is something they can purchase and use at home, once they can use them safely, and know how to avoid injury using them on their own. They are excellent for neuro, cardio and full body workouts.

CHAPTER 22

FINDING A PROFESSIONAL

One of the answers I received when I asked the group of survivors what struggles they face when trying to find a professional to guide them in further recovery was:

They don't know what questions to ask, to know if the professional can help them in stroke recovery.

You probably understand by reading this book that I strongly recommend finding someone who knows the biomechanics of the human body. A caregiver I spoke to said that she wanted to ask the trainers she met what credentials they had, but she felt like it may cause them to be defensive.

If a fitness trainer, Pilates instructor or other fitness professionals have respected credentials and the knowledge to train a stroke survivor, they will be glad to share any information with you that helps you feel comfortable and safe to work with them. If they have experience with survivors, they will understand. Asking to see certifications may not be helpful, since there are many one-day courses as well as quick online certifications.

When I hire a professional yoga, Pilates or fitness/personal trainer to work for me, I have them answer a test on muscles. The knowledge you gained in this book is a good guideline. If you watch them train other people in the gym and it is clear that they are not watching the client's form and or training them in poor form, you know that trainer is not for you. When talking to them, if they don't like answering questions about their education and knowledge to help you, that may mean they don't have it, but do not want to admit it.

Remember that most physical therapists go to college four to six years and many trainers do only a one-day program. Some may continue to get more knowledge. Watching them work and talking to them will show what they know or don't know. I shared some pretty deep knowledge of the body in this book, and I feel every trainer and therapist should understand the body at this level to help a survivor. Specialists who have a college degree in their work would have more knowledge.

I find that anyone who studied under and took courses through Paul Chek and The CHEK Institute has very strong skills and knowledge of working with the body at the level a survivor can really gain from. Pilates instructors who took a large course should be good. Usually they train in hundreds of hours to become a Pilates instructor, although there are a few one-day certifications. I would say if they own a Pilates studio with Reformers, usually that means that they got the solid training. Any physical therapist, personal trainer or studio that understands neurological work should be a good match for survivors.

Whomever you work with, if they have neurological understanding and body mechanics skills and understanding to what a stroke and brain damage is, they should be able to work with a survivor. Athletic trainers usually really understand the movement of the body too. Any of these types of professionals I mentioned should have the ability to keep you safe and avoid injury, as they are working with you.

If you want to be very direct, ask them upfront: *Do you know what the, psoas, multifidus, transverse and pelvic floor muscles are and why they are important in the body?* If they answer with a yes and they actually know, then you probably found yourself a winner. Ask them whatever you need to ask to give you the understanding you need to have to work with them. You can even ask them if they are willing to read this book to help them help you better. Whatever works.

But you have the right to know if they are credentialed and have the proper knowledge to help you. You definitely do not want a trainer faking that they know something, because that is not fair to you. If they continue to talk about how great they are and never let you talk and communicate with you properly, that may not be a good fit either.

In cases where there are limited resources to seek out, keep learning as much as you can, so you can do things on your own. You are going to do things on your own anyway for your daily homework and therapy, so why not understand all that you can.

CHAPTER 23

FINDING SUPPORT GROUPS

When someone has a stroke, it will be life changing for the stroke survivor and their family and caregivers. It can be overwhelming for all involved. There are support groups for survivors and often there are support groups for caregivers as well. For those of you who do Facebook, there are many helpful support groups pages to join. Don't be ashamed or afraid to reach out for mental, emotional and physical help if needed. I included some resources for finding or starting a support group below.

http://www.strokeassociation.org/STROKEORG/strokegroup/public/zipFinder.jsp

http://www.stroke.org/stroke-resources/stroke-support-groups

https://www.flintrehab.com/2018/online-stroke-support-group/

https://www.saebo.com/start-stroke-support-group/

CHAPTER 24

ABOUT THE AUTHOR

Tracy L. Markley has been working and studying in the fitness industry for over 20 years. She is the owner of Tracy's Personal Training, Pilates and Yoga Studio. Previously, she lived in Huntington Beach, California, for 17 years and relocated to Oregon in 2013. She is a Certified Health Fitness Specialist, Personal Trainer, Dance & Group Exercise Leader, Fitness & Nutrition, Biomechanics Specialist, AFAA Group Exercise Examiner, BOSU® Master Trainer, FiTOUR Pro-Trainer, Reiki Master-Teacher, as well as a Pilates and Yoga Instructor. In November 2017, she published her first book, "The Stroke of an Artist,

The Journey of a Fitness Trainer and a Stroke Survivor." An inspiring journey of a stroke survivor. In March 2018, she published her second book, "Tipping Toward Balance A Fitness Trainer's Guide to Stability and Walking." This book is an excellent balance and fall prevention book for seniors. Her third book, "Stroke Recovery What now? When Physical Therapy Ends, But Recovery Continues." This book will be published in November 2018. Her fourth book, "Your Brain, The Software of Your Body, A Fitness Trainer's Guide to Brain Health," will publish in December 2018.

In July 2018, she was asked to be on the Fitness Education Advisory Board for Medfited.org and to write CEC Certification Programs for professionals on "Stroke Recovery and Exercise" and "Back Care and Scoliosis." Tracy is available for speaking events, book signings and training. She can be contacted at her websites
www.tracyspersonaltraining.com and
www.tracymarkley.com
www.instagram.com/motivate_healthyfit

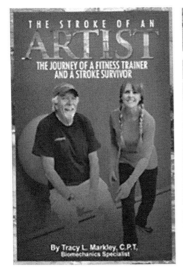
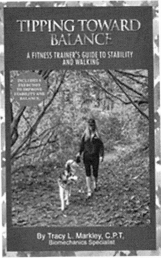
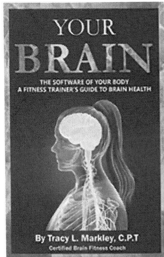
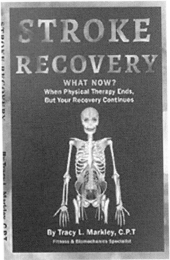

Books available in Paperback, Kindle
& Audio, at Tracy's Websites,
Amazon.com and Audible.com

Made in the USA
Monee, IL
15 January 2020